© Copyright 2007 Christopher Day.
Christopher Day asserts his moral right under the Copyright, Designs and Patents Act, 1988, to be identified as the author of this work.

All rights reserved. No part of this publication may be reproduced, stored in a retrieval system, or transmitted, in any form or by any means, electronic, mechanical, photocopying, recording, or otherwise, without the written prior permission of the author or his representative.

Keywords: Dying, terminal illness, disability, ALS, MND, Lou Gehrig's Disease, teaching the medical profession, autobiography, self-development, self-help, humour.
This book was written with the support of an Academi Writers' Bursary from the Welsh Academy.

Cover design and typesetting by Jeff Bartlett.
Angel legs by Aloma Day.
Illustrations by the author.

Note for Librarians: A cataloguing record for this book is available from Library and Archives Canada at www.collectionscanada.ca/amicus/index-e.html
ISBN 1-4251-0622-6

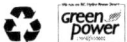

Printed in Victoria, BC, Canada. Printed on paper with minimum 30% recycled fibre.
Trafford's print shop runs on "green energy" from solar, wind and other environmentally-friendly power sources.

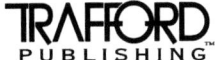

Offices in Canada, USA, Ireland and UK

Book sales for North America and international:
Trafford Publishing, 6E–2333 Government St.,
Victoria, BC V8T 4P4 CANADA
phone 250 383 6864 (toll-free 1 888 232 4444)
fax 250 383 6804; email to orders@trafford.com

Book sales in Europe:
Trafford Publishing (UK) Limited, 9 Park End Street, 2nd Floor
Oxford, UK OX1 1HH UNITED KINGDOM
phone +44 (0)1865 722 113 (local rate 0845 230 9601)
facsimile +44 (0)1865 722 868; info.uk@trafford.com

Order online at:
trafford.com/06-2380

10 9 8 7 6 5 4 3 2 1

Foreword

Dr Susan P Closs, FRCP, FRCPath, Ty-Olwen Hospice

As a consultant in palliative medicine and throughout my medical career, I have witnessed many patients struggle with the knowledge of the imminence of their death. Only very few reach acceptance and inner peace sufficient to both enrich the lives of others around them or to appreciate being rather than achieving.

Death is a taboo subject in our society and many carers avoid entering into a conversation or situation that might lead to facing this issue with their patient or loved one. It is probable that this is partly a reflection of their own inability to acknowledge their mortality. Christopher shows that it is possible to live and to enjoy being, even in the face of a progressive illness.

This book has shed all pretences and is both inspirational and refreshing. Christopher has used humour and the ability to laugh at himself to disclose a vast array of ridiculous situations caused by both his illness and the ineptitude of the health and social care community.

Due to time pressure and other excuses, some professionals do not have opportunity for "conversation" or continued communication with patients who can no longer speak. Others equate physical disability with mental frailty and make no effort at all to communicate.

This book provides insight into a world where even acts, which we do without thought, such as putting on a pair of socks, become a major challenge. The descriptions of the manoeuvres required for daily living remind me of somebody trying to describe a game of cricket and how silly it sounds when put in words. However humorous it sounds when recounted the story affords an important learning platform. We rarely get told (or allow ourselves to hear) the reality of living with disease and become complacent in the fact that "we know best" because we are the so-called experts. Told with such humour and humility, the lessons which Christopher sets out as his own learning points, must be taken on board by the professionals.

Christopher's observations on relationships, particularly about love and the realisation that self worth becomes more important as the body fails are such an important contribution to our understanding of the spiritual domain. It is a poignant reminder of our need to attend to spirituality and not dismiss it to the "too difficult box".

His personality and spirit shine through the experience and the adversity he has encountered. We will all die and I hope that when my time comes I will undertake my personal journey with such good grace and fortitude.

This narrative should be essential reading for all health and social care providers – especially those of us who think we are doing a good job. The gap between our intention and reality for patients is shocking. I am humbled by the author's courage and stoicism and will hopefully use my new found insight and awareness in my practice and in my teaching.

to Oleńka

Acknowledgements

I owe thanks to the many who have encouraged me to write this book, especially nurses, therapists, and patients at Park Attwood Clinic. Also to son, Dewi Day for constructively critical advice and help with the title, and to Nicole van Schie for help tracing publishers. Great thanks are due to Jeff Bartlett for the layout and cover, and to my daughter, Aloma Day for help and support, editorial and cover advice and proofreading. And most especially to Aleksandra Kaczmarek, without whose encouragement, I would never have written more than two or three chapters.

Disclaimer

I do solemnly set down the events, which happened in my declining ears. All events and locations are accurately described, but characters are entirely frictional. Moreover, any sue-able material was not written by me, but by my cat, who has taken to sitting on my computer. It may indeed be true that a monkey left with a typewriter could never write the works of Shakespeare in a million years. (Why would it want to? And anyway, whoever heard of a monkey living a million years?) But (as every cat knows) cats are cleverer.

(my) **Dying is Fun**

A Comedy of Disabled Mis*adventures*

Christopher Day

Contents

An Unchosen Journey
1. Living (or Dying) with a Death-sentence Disease — 1
2. Life before dying — 5
3. (Almost) Coping: a Therapeutic Journey — 17
4. Gadgets and Improvisations — 27
5. Everyday Life: Non-everyday problems — 33
6. Falls — 42

At Home and Elsewhere
7. Beds I have known — 49
8. Chairs I Trust; Chairs I Don't Trust — 56
9. Domestic Staff — 60
10. Bio-hazards: Living with Teenagers and Other Animals — 65
11. Surviving Architecture: non-accessible accessibility — 70
12. Getting to Where to Get Cured: Complimentary Therapy Rooms — 79
13. Places to stay in; Places not to stay in — 84

Moving around
14. Walking Aids — 91
15. Wheelchairs — 98
16. Disabled-unfriendly Cities — 102
17. Public Toilets: Getting In, Getting Out, and Getting to Use Them — 106

Medical and other treatments
18. Hospital Life - or half-life — 115
19. Getting cured, not-cured and fleeced: Assorted Therapies — 120

Officialdom
20. Dealing with the Government — 135

Travelling
21. Trains, planes, boats and me — 138
22. Cars and their drivers — 152

At Work
23. Conferences — 159

Life in General, Death in particular
24. Disabled Love — 164
25. Why Me? Life isn't Fair — 166
26. Last words — 169

An Unchosen Journey

1. Living (or Dying) with a Death-sentence Disease

I always used to think life was an upward journey. At school, they told me to grow up; at college, to pull my socks up; at work, to get up off my... (I think the word was "donkey"). I was then expected to rise in the world. (Something to do with a kick up the donkey?) But I never thought it would involve sitting on clouds. All this changed in just one day. The day I realized I'm mortal. The day I discovered I'm living under a death-sentence. The day I realized that every day is a day nearer death. (That might have always been so, but no-one had told me before.) At least, that's how it felt when I was diagnosed with Motor Neurone Disease (Lou Gehrig's Disease, ALS – I've heard about Lou, but who was Al?). I asked the prognosis and was told "Usually one year. In your case (as diagnosis was difficult) probably several." Frank. Perhaps I would have preferred a little less frankness.

Outwardly calm, but inwardly reeling, I often wondered what "several" meant: more than a couple, less than ten, probably less than half a dozen. Many prisoners on Death Row in US jails get longer. At that, I mentally wrote myself a programme: one year limping, one using a walking stick, one on two sticks, one on crutches, one on a zimmer frame, one in a wheelchair, one in bed, one on a cloud doing harp practice (or - if unlucky - not on a cloud, but *in* a cloud (of smoke), stoking a furnace)

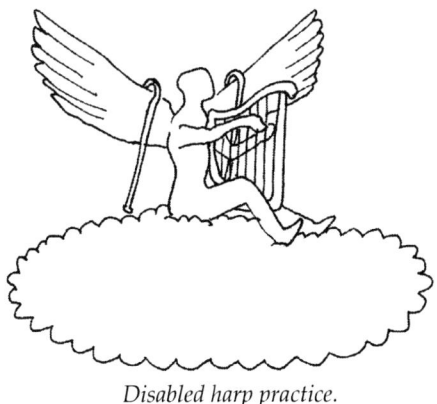

Disabled harp practice.

Unfortunately (for the programme), I'm not good at doing what the government tells me to do. It is now five years, so I'm in the period between two and six years; the "several" year period. I'm not dead, I'm not well, I'm significantly disabled (I walk with crutches and can barely speak) but I've never felt better in my life.

Living (or Dying) with a Death-sentence Disease

Why?

There are three nasty things about terminal illness: pain, fear of death, things going wrong with the body. I'm lucky. No pain. Were I in continual pain, I probably wouldn't think life was fun. Nor am I afraid of death. Of course, I may be deluding myself, but I don't *feel* afraid. Why should I? After all, most people will probably die one day. (Some say all, but I'm cautious about being too categorical about anything.)

I started out by cultivating a stoical attitude. If death was the prognosis, I would just have to live with it. (Or - should I say? - die with it.) Anyway, I would have to live until I died. After that, there wouldn't be much to worry about.

True, death doesn't have to be for ever. If you don't believe in afterlife or reincarnation, you can pay a mere million dollars to be frozen till, at some time in the future, a cure is found. Of course, a cure is no use if you can't pay the medical bills so it would be wise to set aside another million - and still hope that, after inflation, it will buy more than a preliminary consultation. Nor would you want to come back poor, so add another million. This means that just *before* you die (this is important, after is too late!) you and two million dollars get safely frozen. Once frozen, however, your heirs might want to unfreeze the two million dollars. What is to stop them paying a mere thousand to have you unfrozen as well?

Death didn't seem a very appealing prospect. But my attitude changed when I began to meet some living dead: people who had already died – but not successfully; they were still alive. These actually *enjoyed* life – and told me death was even *better*. (I should have known, of course, that mountains go both up and down. Which is better depends on viewpoint. Climbers enjoy going up. Skiers find down more fun.)

The first ex-dead person I met had, as a teenager, been given experimental drugs. (US pharmaceutical companies used to test their drugs in Spain and Greece in those days. Now - I'm told - they use third world countries.) Six of the seven patients so treated died. So did she - clinically. Unfortunately, she wasn't allowed to stay dead. She experienced - as so many others have related - a bright light and the feeling of being enveloped in love. But for her the journey stopped: a gentle voice told her she was not yet ready for death - and she returned to the land of the living. For a long time afterward, she regretted not being allowed to properly die, so blissful was the experience. She also told me not to worry about only being given a year to live. After being told this for nine years, her doctors gave up telling her. After all, it isn't very professional to tell a patient: "I'm sorry you aren't dead. Whoops! I meant: I'm sorry, you aren't dead. No. I really meant: You aren't dead. I'm sorry."

Living (or Dying) with a Death-sentence Disease

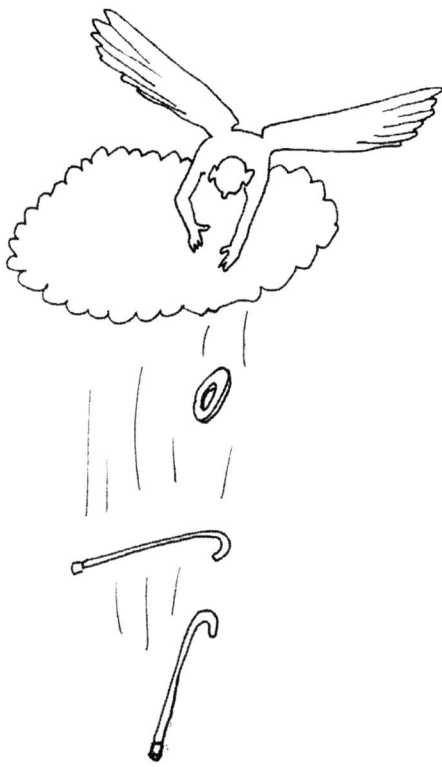

Cloud-sitting errors.

A mere two months later, I met someone else who had died - but she had done it five times (also in hospital, so five-fold professionally verified). Five times sounds like really serious dying practice - so she was really professional at dying and knew all about it. She was anyway a professional: a doctor - and, not surprisingly, an exceptional one, but more of her later.

So much for death. It's going to come one day. Few of us want to accelerate that time, though many of us do so by our chosen lifestyles. As it seems it will be sooner for me, I must hurry to write this book. Hurrying, however, is something my illness has taught me not to even bother trying to do. Life, by necessity, is nice and slow. Anyway, it's slow - and nicer that way; it gives me more chance to *enjoy* life.

Things going wrong is the biggest issue. Lots goes wrong: walking (and falling), carrying things, doing things, breathing and speaking, eating, drinking and peeing; getting dressed, turning over in bed, and more...

Living (or Dying) with a Death-sentence Disease

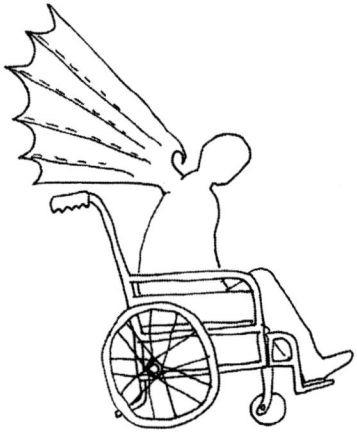

Wrong wings – I hope!

When I first started limping, I hoped no-one would notice, but after a while it wasn't something I could hide. Then came a new symptom: "inappropriate laughter". I not only laughed at inappropriate moments, but made decidedly odd noises when I did so. These were *very* embarrassing. My teenage daughter didn't dare sit beside me in the cinema! Unfortunately, so odd were my choking, gasping and wheezing trying-not-to-laugh noises that I couldn't help laughing at *these*. (Why hadn't they told me I would deteriorate to laughing at myself?) There is a logic here I don't understand: Laughing is a symptom of my illness. Illness is Bad. But laughing makes life more fun. Is it that illness and life don't go together? Does that mean I shouldn't be alive?

Of course there are two approaches to humour in adversity. One is: if you don't laugh, you can only cry. The other is that the world and its happenings really *are* funny. Unfortunately, it's hard to laugh if you only want to cry. Fortunately, it's hard to cry if you can't help laughing.

The trouble is that just about everything can go wrong. Even things that can't go wrong, do when I do them. As I can't help (inappropriately) laughing, these now go even more hilariously wrong. This makes it hard to be too serious about anything. As I can't help laughing at the not-funny, eventually, (almost) everything ends up *being* funny. Not necessarily *easy*, but at least funny - and this is much more important. After all, we can live without an easy life, but what sort of life do we live if it isn't fun?

Perhaps not *everything* is funny. Some things are only funny afterwards. Some very few things, just like life, are never funny. This is a pity, because as long as I continue to resent them, I can't grow. Most things however are so comical – or anyway, odd - that life is better now than it ever was before my illness. It's certainly much more fun. As I'm officially dying (actually, *really* officially, I should be dead), I can only conclude that my dying is fun.

2. Life before dying

I was born, an only child, during the war. Despite close bombs repeatedly blowing out windows and an incendiary in the bedroom, whenever air-raids ended, I would demand "More noise! I want more noise!" - a sentiment not widely shared. This was probably my first lesson in not taking the serious too seriously. My only *actual* wartime memories, however, are my Mickey Mouse gas mask - the rubbery smell put me off Disney for life - and joyfully stamping into a war-related puddle, which horrifyingly turned out to be waist-deep. This may be what led me towards pacifism. War, I learnt, is unpredictable, uncomfortable, dirty, dangerous and wet.

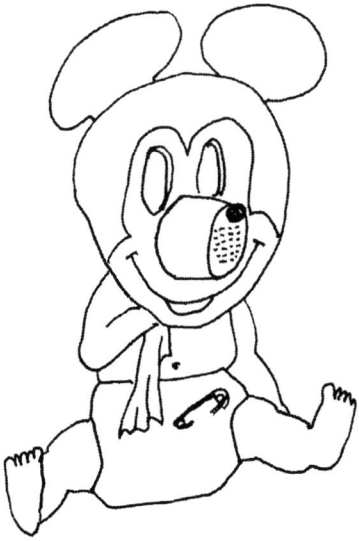

Me, aged one.

When I was seven, my father retired from the army, bought a derelict smallholding and started a market garden - his lifelong dream. Living on a farm, I learnt how to make, repair and improvise things. Money is always short on farms, so resourcefulness is essential. Nor are shops close, so self-reliance is a way of life. From pigs, I learnt the value of logic. Big gaps in fences, like gates, they're clearly meant to go through - but that is the sausage route to heaven. Tiny gaps, they're obviously not meant to go through – but these lead to kitchens and dustbins – heaven on earth.

Also at seven, I was sent to boarding school. Of that school, I have nothing but good memories - obviously the bad ones are too painful to access. Life for me now consisted of two unbridgable halves: school and home. Home life was happy. But school.....

Life before dying

At thirteen I went to another boarding school. This I didn't enjoy. Reinforced by the view that "beating was good for character-development", a culture of sadism ruled amongst the cane-wielding prefects. First-year boys were assigned to them as virtual slaves, called "fags". This taught me to be cautious about revealing my past.

One day a week, we dressed up as soldiers, complete with mirror-polished boots. Being a tiny weed, I looked ridiculous in uniform, but did enjoy playing with real guns - with which, one boy, finding live ammunition, nearly blew his friend's foot off. Also we learnt how to blow-up bridges - a skill useful for blowing-up schools. Although not judged prefect material, a typing error promoted me to corporal. I mentally vowed, however, never to give an order - neither in school, toy-army, nor later life. This was probably the foundation for my career as a consensus-based architect.

From school, I learnt important lessons: Bottle up pain. Separate feeling, thinking and what you do. (All good for a career as a soldier.) Sever body from soul. (What soldiers should do to their enemies.) I also learnt how to love a table - in Latin. This took two years: one to decline love (ammo - also used for shooting friends' feet) and one for table (mensa - something which I later discovered women have). This was my first lesson in love.

All my post-school life, I've been trying to unlearn these lessons - with some success: I can now look at a table without the faintest quiver of desire.

Most of what I learnt at school was either irrelevant or out-of-date. Latin, I learned 1500 years too late. (Had I known that, perhaps *antique* tables might have improved my love life.) The empire wasn't; it was now the commonwealth. (Nor was it really that; the only wealth it owned in common was the Queen - not easily liquefiable into cash.) I did, however, learn French. The first year, we studied être - to be. The following year, however, as preparation for life, we abandoned deep philosophy in favour of materialism: avoir – to *have*. I also learnt some useful phrases. The first – so presumably the most important – were: "Bonjour Madame. Quelle age avez vous?" I never found these effective chat-up lines.

At eighteen, going to architecture school was like release from prison. From now on, any rule - even if I secretly agreed with it - had to be broken on principle. Expect for the mandatory sex (easier to want than to get), drugs (unappealing as I didn't smoke) and rock-and-roll (already going out of fashion), whatever was in fashion, I had to do the opposite. (I had learnt this from pigs.) Anyway, I already knew I would die young, an unrecognized genius, emaciated and impoverished. In the event - which *still* hasn't happened - only this last adjective proved right.

I didn't, in fact, spend my days in college. Romantically wanting to be an 'artist', with beard and sandals, I started evening sculpture classes. I soon found that as all the 'proper' students spent all day in the pub, the tutors were happy if I came by day. Architecture I now did only at night. After three years I got my certificate but, being arrogantly anarchistic, anti-establishment and anti-paper, I never bothered to collect it. (Later, I wanted it, but the college had changed its name and forgotten about me - how humiliating for an unrecognized genius!)

At twenty, I hitch-hiked to Greece and Turkey. Keen to practice my language skills, I asked a German driver: "Soll Ich meinen Gepäck im Hintern stecken?" he looked a little taken aback. Only later did I discover this meant: "Shall I shove my luggage in your behind?" Sleeping out, on my own, in urban-edge waste-ground felt scary, but the only real risks were some of my drivers. These provided an early lesson in trusting in God. Through trying hard to be agnostic, whom else could I trust? It would hardly be wise to trust *their* driving skills!

Surprisingly, I found countries differed most in frontier-regions - where they were nearest each other — but least in capital-city centres - their hearts. Should this have been a lesson for life? Something about hearts despite differences? Certainly, I experienced generosity and warmth unheard of in Britain. I was given lifts by both the Greek and Turkish army - almost at war with each other. Hitching outside a Turkish army base (the only traffic: two trucks per hour), a sentry brought me a chair to sit on. German and Yugoslav policemen stopped vehicles to get me rides. I was housed and fed by both an SS paratrooper and a French Resistance member (separately, thank goodness). This was an early lesson in humanity overriding even the most powerful generalizations. Since then, I've never been able to categorize. This makes filling in forms hard - should I tick *all* boxes, or none?

I then went to work in a big office and got so bored that I swore never to work in an office again. I left to enroll as a 'proper' sculpture student. This diploma I did collect, but being artistically white embossed on white, it didn't make impressive photocopies to apply for jobs with.

After art school, and still not dead, I made sculpture and taught in a London architecture school. Here, I found that architects were more concerned with buildings' *appearance* than how they are to *be* in. Could something be missing? This led to concern for buildings as *environment*, then to how they *impact* environment - obvious, but in those days, revolutionary.

Attending Emerson College, I leant how *underlying* currents shape the world. I also learnt the values of equanimity, patience, dispassionate objectivity, flexibility, appreciation, persistence and compassion. I still find these - especially the first seven ones - hard to practice.

My wife and I then moved back to Wales to build a house. I now discovered how little practical construction I had learnt at architecture school. Indeed, what little I did know, I had learnt on the farm. As an eco-purist, I refused to use machinery, so making hard work inestimably harder. Blending into the landscape with its grass roof, and low-energy with its wind-generator, it wasn't an everyday sort of house, but neighbours liked it and asked me to design extensions, even houses, for them.

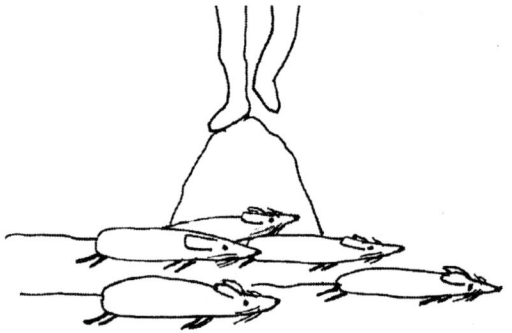

Avoiding the rat-race.

I soon began to get a reputation as a 'green' architect. (Green, in most senses of the word, but not facial colour.) Before I realized it, I had an architectural practice. (Little a because I wasn't a registered Architect.) A friend suggested I apply for registration under a hitherto unused clause. All that was needed was for a committee of at least fifteen board members to approve my application with no more than one dissenting. Fourteen came and unanimously approved - but without a fifteenth to disapprove, I couldn't be accepted! It then took over a year to get a larger committee together. Of thirty, forty, fifty (or whatever) surely two wouldn't approve, but fortunately none did. So now I am legal! And with my own office! So much for swearing I would never work in one again! This taught me to give up swearing.

While building this house, we lived in a 9' x 5' chicken hut wired down against take-off in gales. We were sustained by the warmth of neighbours. One family, in particular, was unstintingly generous despite their poverty. There was no road to their farm; only a stream, doubling as tractor track. To get there meant walking across two fields and a footbridge over the river. Their house was damp, dark, bitterly cold. The one frugal stove - owned, along with any food within reach, by a vicious tom-cat (one of a series named after the great dictators: this one was Stalin) - couldn't compete with the draught from the hole in the front door, big enough for the sheepdogs to walk through unhindered. They had no water indoors, only in the cowshed. Their English was limited: with different inflections "the buggers are having it" could accurately sum up any imaginable situation. With my present speech difficulties, I now use the same technique: "✧✤✞☆✱ |‹› ♥✦▲◆(✳‹✸◆⟩●" covers a wide range of meanings. Here, I learnt to feel at ease and included amongst a social gathering where I understood (then) not one word of the language. A good experience for

Life before dying

Russia and other overseas work. (I now speak Welsh and quickly picked up the two most essential words of Russian: niet (no) and dollar (dollar).)

These friends caused my first near-death experience: They told us there had been TV warnings about Death-cap mushrooms. Symptoms – namely death – didn't emerge for twenty-four hours, but once eaten, there was no cure. They showed us one – kept for safety in a shoe-box, and, for double-safety, held at arm's length. Sure enough (thinking they were horse-mushrooms), we'd just feasted on lots! No symptoms yet, but no cure – just like life! What could we do? The only thing I could think of was go to bed and have a good sleep so I would be refreshed enough to die properly. (Although this would be my last chance to sleep, I didn't find it very easy.) In the morning I woke up – apparently not dead yet. What to do now? The only thing I could now think of was to continue working on the roof. Around coffee-time - and still not dead – a friend came by. "Have you seen the horse-mushrooms?" he asked. "Are you *sure* they're horse-mushrooms?" I didn't want him dead too. "Yes. They're illustrated in my book." I now realized that my valley friends' television only showed snow-pictures – good for stimulating the imagination, but not good for the nerves.

My wife wanted to farm, so we moved from this beautiful, hand-crafted house - a first, if grudging, lesson in Buddhist non-attachment. (Years later, I met a Buddhist monk who specialized in sand mandalas. Each coloured grain placed singly - three weeks of painstaking work. After a ceremony, everything is then scattered to the wind.) For me, this meant another two years of building up a (literally) falling down ruin. (One wall only needed a push to fall over.) This time, however, I had architectural work to fill before-breakfast and after-supper hours. After this, I hoped never to hand-mix concrete again. But this was not to be.

With friends we started a play-group. Looking for premises, we found a derelict school, vandalized, vampire-daubed and wholly uninhabitable. Our aspirations now expanded to a Steiner school, but, having bought the building, we had no money. Appeals failed to raise a penny so we were faced with a stark choice: sell up or start building with no money.

By a mistake, unfortunately never repeated, the non-profit-making playgroup accidentally made a £36 profit. With this we started. After de-vampirising, we could only do jobs - like digging foundations, but not concreting them - that cost no money. The moment we started, however, help and even money came our way from completely unknown sources. Inspiring and humbling to so experience that we were being 'looked after from above' - or so it felt. Goethe's: "Whatever you can do, or dream to do, begin it. There is beauty, power and magic in it." felt never so true.

Over about thirteen years we (mostly I) renovated and extended this school and then built a new kindergarten. No money meant (virtually) no mechanization,

Life before dying

inefficient work sequences, labour-intensive reclaimed materials - and much heavy-labour drudgery. Nor were conditions particularly safe. Fortunately however, we only lost one and a half volunteers. The half-volunteer, half through a ceiling (interesting for the class below). The whole one in the septic tank. Fortunately again, we found him again – and trebly fortunate: it was only full of water.

Volunteers' unpredictable numbers and skills - or lack of both - made work-planning a nightmare. This was hard work, physically, mentally and - with friction inevitable under such pressures - socially. This was exacerbated by being a founder. For community health, I already knew how vital it is that founders quickly withdraw from influence. I had done, but some new teachers, feeling the need to undo what they perceived as 'founder-influence', also tried to undo the volunteer building programme. It not being right to divide the school, I acquiesced. Painful days! But the school, the volunteer building programme and even I survived - if only just!

The kindergarten was a child-revering school, every detail individually hand-made. Apparently, nobody had built anything like this before - anyway, not with unskilled volunteers. To my surprise, it got a lot of publicity and was favorably accepted - even by architects!

I was now working two days a week on the school, five on architecture, as well as the heavier farm-work and endless finishing-off-house tasks. Looking back, I wonder how I did so much. Never watching TV helped – after a while, snow is boring - but there were still pressures on family life. Inevitably, our marriage didn't survive.

Now came black years. Worst of all was when my ex-wife took the children to Ireland. No phone, and for two long periods, no address. Despite some brighter interludes, failed relationships and encounters with manhunters, this was mostly a period of loss: I remember shaking with grief, too weak to stand and not caring whether I lived or died. A dangerous state - I don't recommend it. If it's true about learning from mistakes, I should be a walking (or hobbling) encyclopedia by now. They say you must hit bottom before you can come back up. Poor bottom! Wasn't character-development at school enough?

When I finally got to see my children, they were living in wooden huts, quite primitive but (apparently) happy. (Of their stepfather's alcoholic rages, I knew nothing till they fled their home - disappearing from the world for three months - another black time.) Instead of a toilet there was the electric-cable trench. Fortunately, this was easy to find even under snow, at night. The texture underfoot was unmistakable. Also, once disturbed, there was smell confirmation. Around the huts, vegetation was particularly verdant. Could there be a connection between the trench leading downhill, its contents and trench-filling

Life before dying

Irish rainfall? This way I learnt relationships are more significant than single things - or people.

In those days, I hardly travelled further than (long) walking distance. (Anyway I preferred walking to driving. Up to three miles, if something isn't worth the extra half-hour each way, it isn't worth going to.) I was also too busy to have contact with news and fashions. (This being the 1970s and 80s, perhaps I was fortunate?) All this changed overnight in 1991 following the publication of *Places of the Soul*. Into this book, I had distilled everything I knew about how places affect us - the fruit of a lifetime of observation, research and feedback from design, illumined by my sculpture background and practical building experience. Being one of the first books about ecological architecture and highly critical of establishment architects, I was surprised how well it was received.

Out of the blue, I was appointed visiting professor in Queen's University, Belfast. Suddenly, I found being a professor meant people hung on my every word, however much drivel. Previously, however well thought-out whatever I said, nobody took it seriously. Like my attraction to bombing but fridgidity towards tables, it was always too different from the acceptable norm.

Suddenly also, work took me across the world - to twenty countries (twenty-two if you agree Texas and Quebec are independent) from California to Siberia. Unlike walking, things can go wrong with long-distance travel. Walking, the worst that can happen is getting lost, at night, in heavy rain, in a field with a bull in it. Here, you can hope the bull is also lost. Not so flying. No bulls - although, on Aeroflot planes, there were calves. Late planes can cause problems: from digestive - supper at 6 a.m., breakfast at 5 p.m. - to bedlessness. Arriving late at Copenhagen after blizzard delays, I found the university (containing my room key) locked. In Ohio (after two days' travel) I arrived to *not* find the person meeting me. I did have his university phone-number, but this too was shut. In Florida, there was no public transport to my destination city (population 100,000) ninety miles away. 'Everyone' - actually six people out of ten - has a car. (Even before the New Orleans floods, those without cars didn't count.) The arranged taxi didn't come. Nor, two hours later (ninety miles plus inefficiency time) did its replacement. A further two hours later, the new office shift knew nothing about it and cared even less. With plenty of money, such problems would be trifling. Not, however - as most of my work was for not-for-profit bodies - on a zero budget. These were good lessons in pairing quick-thinking resourcefulness with absolute calm; survival initiative with patient acceptance. Unfortunately, I always thought too slowly. Fortunately, I usually compensated with impatience.

None of these however, prepared me for Russia.

On my very first day, I learnt the value of careful observation. The passport control officer checked my passport details meticulously. Name: Day – he looked

Life before dying

me up and down: did I look like a day? Eye-colour: "hazel"(what does that mean: leaf, bark, nut?) – he looked me up and down: did I *look* barking nuts? Height: 5' 8" – he again looked me up and down: was I *really* 51811 millimeters? Sex – yet again he carefully looked me up and down (a bit *too* carefully for comfort): *did* I look like a transvestite? (Well, I *hope* that was what he was looking at.) And so on.... After twenty minutes, I had passed inspection and he let me through. My conclusion: he couldn't read English.

Nothing works in Russia; restaurants close for lunch (although saving staff wages, nobody understands why they can't make a profit); concrete bits routinely fall off multi-storey buildings; and apartments have double layers of anti-bandit doors, seven locks between them - one of which is sure not to unlock when you need it. (Hence I've been locked *in*, when due to give a lecture; and *out* when needing to collect my luggage for a plane.)

Much of Russia is ugly - crumbling grey concrete tower-blocks with foot-wide cracks dribbling mastic. It's all dirty - millions of square-miles of industrial haze; streets, their lampposts stolen, potholed and littered with broken vodka bottles. (Streets used to be cleaned each year on Lenin's birthday – but since the fridge keeping his brain broke down, he's no longer able to think about this.) One relief: strewn around Moscow's Park of Culture, a collection of gigantic supine Lenins, Stalins and heroes of the KGB pointing the way forward. (They now point downward – actually, through the ground. Is this a lesson for life?). But I loved Russia. I met - especially in Siberia - a human warmth beyond imagination in the West.

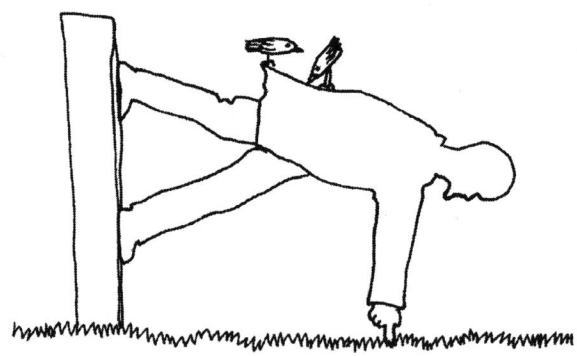

The heroic way downward.

Life before dying

Nonetheless, none of this prepared me for Ukraine. In Crimea, to save water, it only ran from six to eight - and *did* run: where I stayed, there was neither tap nor plug. Also electricity went off at dusk, plunging the town into darkness and leaving us to grope our way around our accommodation, tripping over the dog in the process. This also silenced the sea-front discos just as clubbers arrived - another inexplicably failing business venture. The town was anyway quiet; I only ever saw two trucks, three cars and a bus that could only start downhill. Here I learnt how rich I am; how easy *my* life is! I also learnt that logic is not essential to life; vodka seems an adequate replacement.

Even this, however, didn't prepare me for problems *between* Russia and Ukraine. I had both Russian and Ukrainian visas, but not - as I discovered - permission to *re*-enter Russia after four days in Ukraine. The border guard ordered me off the train. My Russian friend said, "Don't! Let's talk this out." Was there a fine (bribe) to pay? No: unaccountably, the man was honest. She told him I was an important professor, needed for important work in Moscow, couldn't there be a way? Eventually, he agreed to phone a superior and disappeared - with my passport - leaving an armed guard to ensure I did *not* get off the train. During this hour, I had visions of walking along the Russio-Ukrainian border, then the Belarus-Ukrainian, Polish-Ukrainian and Polish-Czech borders till I reached the Czech-Austrian one. Quite a long walk. For this I would need a good breakfast. No food in no-man's land (no-men eat no meals) - and, I rather hoped, no mines. Feeling it appropriate to look calm, I tried to finish breakfast, but this - garlic chicken and bread - required use of my friend's impressively big flick-knife (her Moscow street-defence; pepper-spray is less reliable – if held the wrong way round it's counterproductive). So - no breakfast. Half my brain was making survival plans, the other half thinking "This can't be happening to me. Surely God will look after me." He evidently did, for an hour later, the officer came back, full of smiles and I was allowed to stay on the train. Loud sighs of relief! Time now to open the Crimean brandy, then fetch boiling water from the corridor boiler for tea to soothe our brandy-burnt throats!

Different climates, different cultures, different adventures. But the main thing all this taught me was that whenever I arrived somewhere new, I knew nothing. (Actually I never knew *nothing*. From a test-yourself book, I found I had an IQ of two, which I have since proudly increased to four. It should really be five, but some questions have trick answers. For instance: 'Which is the odd one out: Elephant, kangaroo or table?' Obviously it should be kangaroo – the only one with two legs – but the book gives another answer. I challenge anyone who says I'm stupid to double their IQ so dramatically! I now base my design method on knowing nothing - this lets me ask questions (especially silly ones - which often elicit the most useful answers).

Life before dying

Working in California turned everything I knew upside down. Most of my previous work had been rural; this was ten acres of mixed-use urban development. Commitment to sustainability provided the only continuity, but even here, there were economic and social issues as well as ecological ones - symbiotically interlinked. Moreover, instead of designing buildings against cold and wind, these must defy heat and *induce* cooling draughts. Nobody walked, only drove. Street community didn't exist - indeed, public space wasn't sociable, but dangerous. Saturday nights meant gunshots.

Later, when working to consensually design a yoga camp, I was able to learn enough yoga to stand on my head and really see the world upside down. This made things much clearer. My clients gave me a book called 'Yoga Made Easy'. The cover illustration showed a man in knots. Nowhere, however, did it tell how to *undo* knots. Evidently, these weren't easy. I wondered: was this a lesson for life - is it that only I can undo my own knots?

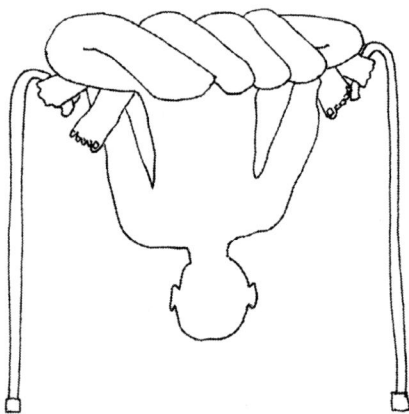

Disabled yoga.

This tied in with what little I know of karma. According to Steiner (if I understand correctly), we are spiritual beings. But not fixed beings; we need to grow, develop. We can't do this sitting on clouds polishing halos. To grow, we need real challenges, obstacles - things, people, situations. Hence we need to incarnate into bodies; to live - and die - in a material world. Our higher-self - or guardian angel - seeks out the particular challenges, growth-opportunities, we need. But growing can be hard work: it often hurts or doesn't serve our egotistical wishes - so we avoid these challenges. But we can't escape the *need* to resolve these issues, situations, aspects of ourselves - so they're re-presented in different forms throughout life, even in subsequent incarnations. We can't evade these issues, but - before we're allowed onto clouds - must face them. Sometimes the only way is through illness.

Life before dying

My second marriage, despite a sunny start, was disastrous and brief. I should have learnt from yoga that everything looks the other way up, once it's upside-down. The bleakness of its finish hit my health. Already ill, I fell and broke my rib - directly over the heart - and promptly followed that with pleurisy, then bronchitis. In those days, living *wasn't* fun. I hadn't realized I was dying. (Nobody had yet told me that we all are.)

Once I actually knew I was dying, I raced to finish my life-work book: *Spirit & Place*. Into this I crammed everything I knew. (Of course I'd done this with *Places of the Soul*, but since then I had lived even longer, reflected longer, and now had twelve years of multi-climate, multi-culture experience, informed by professorial research behind me - fortunately this didn't affect the size of my behind.) Anyway, as a Gemini with a split-childhood, why shouldn't I have two life-works? Indeed, as an only child, why shouldn't I have anything I want?

As it happened, I didn't die - and still haven't yet. (Anyway, it's now too late to die a young genius - so why bother?) Nonetheless, under pressure of dying, I realized that some things I do are unique. Some - like my unique speech - aren't worth recording. My uniquely malfunctioning private functions definitely shouldn't be. But others, like my consensual design approach, should be. Architects are trained to have brilliant ideas – but one person's brilliant idea is someone else's nightmare. Whereas brilliant nightmare-ideas can lead to fights, *condensing* design is innately consensual - even, as I experienced, with a multi-faith, multi-cultural group. 'All' it needs is to leave ego-baggage behind - simple only in theory! This technique - based on what a project needs to 'say', and building upon the place's characteristics, past and future biography, soul and spirit - I hurried to write down as *Consensus Design*.

Life, in short, has been hard work. As I've always believed in what I was doing, I've generally enjoyed this. (Hand-mixing concrete excepted; but fortunately disability gets me out of this). But, as I learnt at school, life *between* work was different: for much of my life, *not* much fun. In the black years I was often depressed. But many, many people have lives incomparably harder than mine. Why aren't they more miserable? Or is miserableness an attitude – nothing to do with how hard life is? In which case, why not choose happiness? That's an attitude too.

One day, I decided I had had enough of being depressed - no longer would I suffer being victim to feeling low. I realized it's nobody's job but my own to feel sorry for me. This gave new meaning to "God helps those who help themselves" (despite the rider: "But God help those who get caught helping themselves"). Life may be unfair, but even less fair was to inflict this on others. Also, once I realized criticism is negative, doesn't help anybody, I decided it was time to stop despising myself whenever I did things wrong. Thereafter, at any mistake, I would now think: "Drat! Silly me! There I go again! How can I do better next time?" Self-acceptance made life much lighter than self-criticism - also, without self-indulgent misery, I could better focus on improving my ways. Why didn't I think of this sooner? (If only I had managed an IQ of five!)

So much for a change of attitude. Once I started dying, however, this brought entirely new challenges. Instead of abstract philosophizing, things just went wrong – very wrong, repeatedly wrong. But, strangely, life became more fun. Perhaps learning to see the world upside down helped. Or is it that for anything to be fun, things *need* to go wrong? Disability makes me good at that.

3. (Almost) Coping: a Therapeutic Journey

My illness has developed slowly. So have my disabilities. Fortunately, these didn't all appear at once; only one new thing goes wrong at a time. Unfortunately, the newest to emerge is always something I just can't cope with - until something else goes wrong and I realize how easy (by comparison) the last problem had been.

Initially, I found limping, falling, and clumsiness embarrassing. But as soon as I could cope with these, I developed sneezing. I just couldn't cope with this. Sneezing may sound inconsequential, but it isn't sociable. It's also dangerous for the person I am talking to. My sneezes are uncontrollable, violent and wet. Moreover, if I've just eaten, there are food bits too - an unfortunate waste. Naturally I politely turn away from anyone near me, but my body jerks back to frontal posture at the key point of the sneeze. So, unless they duck, they get a wet face. If they do duck, they only get a hair wash. As they can't see the food bits decoratively topping the head, I feel it wouldn't be polite to upset them by mentioning these.

Curiously, sneezing while eating seems to lower my popularity. Few people say "Bless you". Most appear to think the opposite. Some don't actually curse me; they just look disgusted and wipe their faces.

Lesson to be learnt: don't talk and eat. Further lesson to be learnt: Don't be ill and ill (cold and MND/ALS) at the same time.

Additional lesson to be learnt: sitting opposed to friends is rude; sitting beside them is more sociable.

After I got used to this, I could cope with everything else, but not incontinence. This *is* embarrassing. It's very embarrassing to wet khaki trousers then stand in front of 300 people to lecture. Only by concentrating solely on what I had to say could I cope with it. Still, no doubt my audience remembered the lecturer, if not the lecture!

As I got slower, incontinence got worse. Usually, I would just get to the toilet in time, no time to shut the door, but then before I reached the receptacle... Totally soaked trousers aren't embarrassing - they're humiliating. Pale trousers show pee conspicuously, but even dark ones go darker when wet. This led me to black trousers.

The next step was to wear nappies (diapers). These are convenient, but do have some disadvantages. As they fill - and over-fill - quickly, I seek every opportunity to pee conventionally. Nappies aren't easy with 'man-trap' toilets - the kind where the seat won't stay up but falls like a guillotine when you least expect it. I need one hand to hold the nappy out of the way, one to direct aim and one to hold back the seat to prevent amputation. I may look and sound odd, but I'm not three-handed. So, which hand can I dispense with? If the first hand,

I will pee in my trousers; if the second, I will pee all over the wall; if the third, I will never pee again. Such toilets put me off women's lib.

As incontinence got worse, the nappies got bigger - hence embarrassingly bulkier. The maximum size - the size I felt most secure with - can absorb one litre. That is to say, if you carefully trickle water all over its whole area, it will hold one litre. My anatomy is not so diffuse. If I jet unmentionable liquid at one point, the nappy rapidly overfills and overflows. As the jet is rarely symmetrically aligned, overflow is usually long before full capacity is reached, hence copious. But even when they don't overflow, nappies aren't problem-free. One litre weighs over two pounds - almost the weight of a brick. My underpants are not designed to carry bricks. The waistband (usually) holds, but the brick works its way through the leg-hole, falling on my foot with a publicly audible squelch. It then unrolls across the floor. In a crowd, you can hope there are too many legs to see feet, and that by looking around disapprovingly, I could pretend the noise came from a neighbour - just as I could with an indiscreet fart. But I daren't stand so close to people lest they trip over my crutches and bring me down. This means embarrassment is unavoidable.

Lesson to be learnt: avoid bricks in trousers.

The inadequacy of nappies led me to sheaths and leg-bags. In effect, I am now a walking (actually hobbling) plumbing system. Plumbing only works if all joints fit tightly. Consequently, what plumbers innocently term male and female components must be sized accurately. (Having seen plumbing-trade calendars, however, I'm not fully convinced all plumbers are so innocent.) To ensure leak-free joints, therefore, convene sheathes come with a penis sizing gauge. The sizes are: small, medium, standard, large, and extra-large. 'Small' is the diameter of my little-finger, so safely pre-pubescent. All the other size names are non-threatening for the male ego. Had a marketing psychologist been involved, however, the gauge would start with pencil-diameter 'cute' and pen-diameter 'standard' (neither manufactured), then progress through 'large', 'extra-large', mega-huge', 'gigantic' and 'elephantine'.

The pee-bag fastens to my leg with two Velcro straps. Simple as these are in principle, their tension isn't easy to get right. If secured too tightly, they tourniquet my leg. This risks gangrene and a lost foot. If they're too loose, the full bag slides down my leg and ankle until I'm hanging a brick off something never designed for hanging bricks. Also it's now so low I can tread on it. This risks a burst bag. Which is worse: loosing a foot or private distortion and public embarrassment?

(Almost) Coping: a Therapeutic Journey

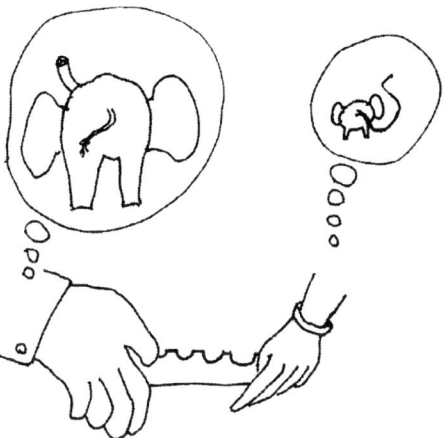

Penis sizing is open to psychological interpretation.

Mostly, however, this system works well - at home. At home I have a bucket to drain the bag into, which I then empty into the toilet. But in town? Here, there are only public toilets - and as I can't get my foot high enough to empty the bag into them and there are no floor-drains, what can I do except hold a lamppost and pretend the puddle had been left there by a dog? As this isn't very sociable, hygienic or even legal, it means travel is still not problem-free.

Sheaths and leg-bags sound like the answer to all problems - but even here, there are snags. The sheath is like a condom with a tube outlet (rendering it useless for black market resale to underage teenagers). Being a 'unique strapless design' (What, I wonder, did the strap secure to? And was it leather or rubber?), it relies on glue. The first sheaths I had, used something akin to superglue. Reassuringly secure by day, but half-an-hour (or more!) of agony to remove at night.

No doubt there were complaints, if not personal injury law-suits, for the Mark 2 sheaths now use a more willy-friendly glue. Painless - unless they catch hairs! These likewise are painless, indeed unfelt, until I fill my bag - also one litre. This pulls them into tension so now I have to walk around with a brick hung off my pubic hair. This is not painless. Fortunately this can be remedied. All it requires is a pocket-knife, courage - and privacy. Invariably, however, I'm in a public place where unzipping, fiddling - and, worse, inserting a knife, might raise eyebrows. Furthermore, few people feel confident being operated on by a spastic surgeon who can't even keep his balance. Nor do I.

There are also plumbing problems. Occasionally the outlet tap snags on my trousers and opens. This isn't only embarrassing, but can also be socially isolating. On one occasion, I found myself marooned in the middle of a lake.

(Almost) Coping: a Therapeutic Journey

Wet floors being lethally slippery for crutches, all I could do was stand still and hope to be rescued.

Joints can also come loose. Fortunately, they don't often. Even more fortunately, they only do so when the bag is at least half full. Or sometimes there is a twist in the sheath. Twists slow flow, so increase water-pressure. Water-pressure isn't good for push-fit plumbing. I never was a good plumber. Invariably, I would find I needed one special part at four on Friday afternoon, just when builders' merchants close. In carpentry, you can make whatever part you need. In plumbing, you can only wait till Monday morning with much gnashing of teeth. It must be karma that I am a pee-plumber now.

Lesson to be learnt: Gnashing teeth builds up a store of embarrassment later.

After I got used to this, I could cope with everything else, but not regurgitation. Sometimes this is just stomach-acid which burns my throat so I can't talk - or even, for a while, can't breathe as breathing fans flames into my windpipe. More usually, I just regurgitate recent food or drink. Cows enjoy this. I don't. It can be quite revolting - especially if it's the remains of an indigestibly unpleasant meal. This has led me to appreciate (savour is too strong a word!) nicer tasting regurgitations.

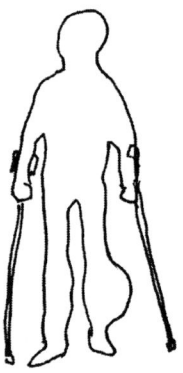

With a urine bag, nobody could ever know I'm incontinent.
They merely think I have a (variable) deformity.

Usually I keep my mouth shut. This is polite and sociable, but I don't always do it. One disadvantage is that if I'm breathing in, I can breathe in recent repast and choke. This is not a good way to enjoy food. Fortunately the district nurse lent me a suction pump. Unfortunately this has a short lead, so I must be careful only to choke near an electrical socket. With the pump come two suction nozzles. One is for sucking through the mouth. And the other one: which opening is that to suck from?

Sometimes my mouth is open. This lets everything slosh out - as much a surprise to any companion as it is for me. This is a good way to loose friends.

(Almost) Coping: a Therapeutic Journey

Being so unpredictable, with not even half-a-second's warning, regurgitation can be nerve-wracking if I'm working on an architectural drawing or book illustration. Weeks of work wasted - and breakfast wasted too! Sometimes I think the world isn't fair.

Occasionally, however, my mouth is only slightly open. This is worst. Like putting a finger over a hose nozzle, power increases a hundred-fold. This can be dangerous for the person I'm speaking to. It also makes me nervous of talking to important people as the more important they are, generally the less humorous. But even amongst humorous people, very few seem to enjoy my breakfast - or anyway, not hour-old breakfast.

Lesson to be learnt: it's considered polite to keep my food to myself. Better for me, better for my friends - and much more economical.

After I got used to this, I could cope with everything else, but not poor speech. Speaking is hard work - and slow. Often I have to repeat things three or four times before I'm understood. This is a disadvantage. Slowness, however, is an advantage. It gives me plenty of time to think - hence good opportunity to pretend to be wise.

Another aspect of slowness is that I often miss the chance to say something. Mostly, this doesn't matter, but occasionally it's important. My memory isn't good, so to remember whatever it was until the next day, I must use technique. I repeat the whatever-it-was to myself in at least four different ways: different words, different grammar, different languages. This usually works – as long as I can remember the translation.

In many ways, not being able to speak is the hardest, certainly the most frustrating, of all my disabilities. But it's also the greatest gift. Every word is such hard work - both to enunciate and for someone else to understand - that I need to choose words carefully, shorten sentences, and be sure that anything I say is worth the effort. Indeed I often conclude that my thought isn't worth saying, so choose silence over speech. In short - and it must be short - I am forced to refine whatever I say to the essential minimum. This doesn't mean that *I* am refined, but it does ensure that I don't waste anyone else's time with things not worth saying. (Actually, I already knew that brevity sells newspapers. Two words are all a headline needs. 'SEX SHOCK' – or variations like 'SHOCKING SEX', 'SEXY STOCKING – suffice for any newsworthy story. I just hadn't learnt that brevity is also applicable to life.)

Not being able to do things myself, but having to rely on verbal instructions, has taught me that even simple statements are open to wide ranging interpretations. When, at a group table, I asked "Can you push my chair in please.", the responses were varied:

"He wants to be moved to the side."

"Turn him this way."

(Almost) Coping: a Therapeutic Journey

"He wants his plate filled."

Most listeners were mostly correct: I *did* want something. But one was strikingly novel. "Where did you say you lived dear?" I didn't know my speech was *that* bad! "I'm a little bit deaf." What a relief - I hoped this was an understatement!

Some people never understand me. They *think* they understand - and that is the problem. Once they 'know' what I'm saying - often totally opposite to what *I* think I'm saying - every time I repeat it, their 'understanding' is confirmed. This leads to exchanges like:

"Could you pass the milk please."

"You want some prunes?"

"No! Milk."

"How many, dear?"

"I don't want prunes."

"I agree. I always have them too - keeps everything running smoothly."

'Things' running smoothly is exactly what I do *not* want. My legs can't run, so what can I do if anything else wants to? But anyway, what can I do? I have to learn to accept whatever life brings. Even if this is prunes - and their consequences.

In such communication impasses I eventually have to accept whatever *they* think I said. Indeed, accept it or not, as I have, in their ears, said it four times, I have no understandable argument to counter this. This continually reminds me of a dentist who, whenever he had the drill safely at work in my mouth, used to tell me what I believed in and did. I didn't and didn't. In the circumstances, however, it seemed wise not to deny it.

Interestingly, to those who can't understand me, naughty Voice gives up at the third attempt. Non-understanders generally either don't listen or are so fixed in what they think they've heard they can't entertain other possibilities. So even if they did understand my speech, they wouldn't hear what I said. Hence: why bother? Voice seems to know this better than I do.

Lesson to be learnt: 'knowledge' blinds listening observation.

Further lesson to be learnt: It's just not worth talking to people who won't listen.

Political lesson to be learnt: Only vote for politicians with speech impediments. It isn't worth their while saying anything not worth saying. Totally dumb ones are best. (True, some world leaders are totally dumb, but ones who can't speak are safer.)

When my speech is too bad, nobody understands so I draw pictures, write words or use hand signals. For brevity, I edit hard, so just write the keywords of what I want to say, like 'book on shelf 2 U.' This frequently results in blank expressions. Obviously most people are used to full sentences, so I have to then add the preceding part of the sentence. There being no space in the appropriate part of the paper, this now reads: 'book on shelf 2 U I want 2 give.' This covers all the essential information, but unfortunately, not everyone is used to understanding life backwards. (Was it worth giving them a book?)

There is also the small problem that few people can read my writing, and even less can read it upside down. They ought to, because turning the paper usually means I drop it. That's why I prefer drawing. It's also quicker. And, as is widely said: " a picture is worth a thousand words." Some people, however, have a vocabulary of less than one thousand words. (For a pub conversation, you only need six hundred. Indeed, when you reach the stage of maximum fluency, ten will suffice.) For sub-thousand-worders, two pictures are a thousand words too many. There are also a surprising number of people who are too used to a verbal world; expecting to read words, they don't even understand pictures. When I drew bookshelves to show where something was, one person tried to read each shelf-line as a word. Inexplicably, she couldn't.

Lesson to be learnt: you can't make everyone happy, all the time. You can't make everyone understand, all the time. You can't make some people understand, any of the time.

When all else fails, hand signals are the most unequivocal. For normal daily life you only need a few: thumb up for "yes" or "good"; thumb down for "no" or bad", and fingers to count with. As my better arm only rotates about sixty degrees, there isn't much difference between good and bad - just like life. Also, many unobservant people can't tell the difference - again, like life. Unfortunately, some people like to ask double questions like: "Would you like this one? Or this one?" You can't answer this with a simple affirmative thumb, so I sign "one" or "two" with my fingers. With limited arm rotation, my palms face me when putting fingers up. One slight problem is that some people take offence at the number one, as communicated by finger. Some even get offended by the number two.

Lesson to be learnt: communication is always open to misinterpretation.

Further lesson to be learnt: people only hear what they expect - even if I use finger gestures for clarity.

(Almost) Coping: a Therapeutic Journey

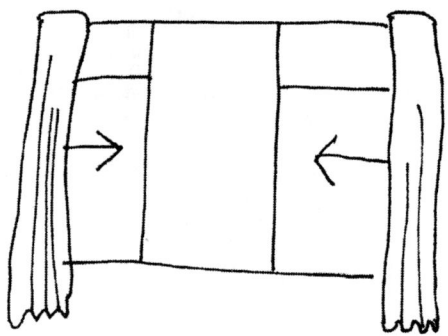

This drawing meant to say: "Please close the curtains."
But the nurse answered: "Which book do you want?"
At last I understand why the Bible says:
"In the beginning was the word." Not: "In the beginning was the pictures."

Finger gestures are fine for one-word answers, but more complicated questions require richer answers. T for tea is easy to gesture with the hands. But milk? For this I resort to hand-milking movements. What could be clearer? (I do, however, omit the bucket clenched between my thighs. This could open the way to more serious misunderstandings.) Likewise, when a nurse, asking about my sleep, didn't understand when I said the dawn birds wake me, I had to resort to whole-body gestures. I thought this would help, but from her expression, she understood even less. In fairness, I doubt many of her patients flap their arms and extend their noses with finger and thumb making tweeting motions. Apparently, this was not the answer she had been expecting.

So much for simple statements. What about complicated sentences involving things like: chilies, digestive disturbance (without being rude), and Australians (remember: I can't stand on my head)? This strains my powers of mime and can produce very interesting expressions on my listeners' (actually: watchers') faces. Also, some words like "tea-break" are easy to gesture (T and break), but easily misunderstood (I never wanted broken tea). Sometimes, I realize, it's better not to say anything. A lesson I should have learnt years ago.

If talking is hard, telephoning is even harder. My survival skills, like drawing pictures and making hand gestures, don't seem to help. Worst of all is ringing a business in London. London seems to run faster than where I live, and I'm slow anyway. Often it goes like this: ring, ring, ring, "Hello?" Having breathed out during the rings, I now have to take a breath to speak. This gives just enough time for the other person to say three more hellos and put the phone down. Sometimes they're so speedy that they start (what they assume is inaudible) swearing before their handset has quite reached its cradle. I try again. Repeat - and rather more swearing. When I do eventually get to speak, most people don't understand me. They know I'm drunk - they can hear how I slur words, and I've already tried to irritate them, which *they* don't think funny. (Few ask whether I do.) Anyway, they're busy and have much more important things to do than wait for me to breathe.

Often they ask me to repeat something. I take a breath and try again. The more forbearing ones suggest I get someone else to speak to them. I try, therefore, to call someone else in the house; I shout "Hello". From the phone comes "Hello". "I'm trying to call someone to speak to you." "Can you call someone to speak to me?" "I'm trying to." "Will you call someone!" I turn away from the phone and shout "Hello". "Hello" from the phone and our non-conversation starts all over again.

Unfortunately, my bad language can upset people in ways I never intended. When staying at a clinic and just about to telephone a friend, the phone rang. Remarkable! Telepathy! But it wasn't my friend. An unknown voice said "How are you darling?" Wracking my brains as to who this could be, I asked who was speaking. Answer: "Paul, you do sound bad." "I'm not Paul." "Darling, I'm so sorry." "I'm not Paul. I'm Christopher." "Don't worry, darling, I understand. I hope you'll soon be feeling better. I can tell from your voice how low you are." It's difficult to disengage from a conversation when whatever you say gets you further onto the hook. All I could offer was many "good-byes" - none of which were understood - and put the phone down. At least, however, I did discover that even strangers know that I am low, and also that Paul was bad - though whether 'interesting' or criminal, I didn't know.

Bad language isn't good for work. Once potential clients hear my voice, they quickly decide they don't want to talk to a drunkard and hang up. With those I have to ring back, it's even worse. While I was struggling to speak, one woman thought I was a 'breather'. So far, however, I've evaded the police - or perhaps they just can't think of a way to interview me?

What's the point of answering phones if no-one understands me? I realized I should try to learn few essential words - one each week. The first – and most invaluable – was "NO". In any situation, this is a safe answer, so qualifies me for any job. Next, I learnt "DON'T". A vital defensive word, this is always useful, and would guarantee my safety from any misguided help. Next came "I". This lets me personalize all communication. These three words suffice for all needs, spanning as they do from "NO" through "I DON'T KNOW" (true practically all the time) to "AYE". I therefore felt no need for any more, so stopped learning in case I wore out my brain.

Speaking badly, however, does have some advantages: I have a good excuse to not answer the phone and PVC window salesmen get fed up talking to me. (Actually I don't need an excuse - if the phone is out of reach I can't get to it in time). Mostly, however, bad speech - like bad language - is a disadvantage.

I can cope with all this, even not speaking, but the worst thing of all

(Almost) Coping: a Therapeutic Journey

is dependency. Having to depend on people who don't care is wearing. Depending on people who *do* care is even worse. I become a burden they would never give up. This is not a good thing to do to other people. But I have no choice. Or have I?

Before I became ill, I used to do too much. Working, building, single-parenting; growing food, volunteer projects, lecturing, writing - every waking minute. Fortunately, I enjoyed everything I did. Some people have to do as much but hate it. Nonetheless, it was too much. What could I give up? Anyone who has been in this position knows the answer: nothing. There was, however, an alternative: get ill. I now can do hardly anything. Just as bad speech has forced me to learn to edit hard and *not* say things, so does incapacity force me to prioritize and not do things. I also have to learn to prioritize and limit what I ask of others.

Alternatively, I could look forward to the next thing to go wrong - something new not to cope with; something to make all previous problems seem bearable.

4. Gadgets and Improvisations

Things you can buy

Life is disabled–unfriendly. This means you need gadgets to make things easier. Many you can buy - for these, there are catalogues. As I don't speak well, I need a gadget to help me. The hospital kindly lent me one. It's quite simple: a microphone and amplifier, but quite complicated - lots of wire to get tangled round my neck. All I have to do is put on a head-grip that looks like earphones, then adjust the microphone in front of my mouth, plug in all leads and clip the amplifier box to my belt.

There are, however, complications.

Firstly, the head-band looks so like earphones that people shout at me. But I'm not deaf. Being slow, there are delays while I switch on the amplifier, then take a breath to speak - but now can't because the other person is shouting louder... So I take another breath and...

When I eat, the microphone is in front of my mouth. This requires skilled fork control. And even more skilled spoon control for if spoons bump, they capsize, tipping soup onto my chest. Spaghetti is even worse. It easily tangles around the microphone with interesting acoustic effects. I now understand why it is rude to talk while eating.

But there are more problems. When I sit, the amplifier slides up off my belt. When I stand, it falls between my legs, suspended from the wire round my neck. This makes it hard to speak. It isn't even easy to walk as when the amplifier swings back and forth it hits me in a place that isn't very comfortable.

Fortunately, all problems can be overcome. Instead of clipping the amplifier to my belt I can clip it to my pocket edge. There is only one slight drawback. My voice now emanates from my crotch. Not all respectable people find this appropriate. Whether or not it's true that all men think from the crotch, it's not normally considered polite to speak from it. Not to mention the odd noses I make when I laugh.

Lesson to be learnt: think where you are speaking from.

Fortunately, I now have a better device. This has a throat microphone which clips around the neck; also a strap to hang the amplifier round my neck. The microphone is sensitive. It broadcasts every swallow, every breath. This means I am always assured of an audience, but even so it doesn't help self-confidence. Even more embarrassing are the sounds of eating. Another reason not to speak while eating.

A neck-strap amplifier is a great improvement over a crotch-mounted one. But when I walk the amplifier swings back and forth hitting me in the chest. The resulting hollow slap travels up my windpipe to the throat microphone, then down the wires to the amplifier. Still, this is better than the noises I make

Gadgets and Improvisations

when struck by an amplifier between the legs.

To avoid this, I hang the amplifier over my shoulder. Being heavy, it quickly slides down to under my armpit. This also is an odd place to speak from, but less rude. Putting on a pullover adds further complications - so many wires and strings. Hence I put it on over the appliance. Consequence: muffled armpit voice.

Lesson to be learnt: technology can solve all things - but how? Is there such a thing as a clean technology?

Further lesson to be learnt: try and keep speech clean.

When my speech deteriorated further, all the amplifier could do was amplify my bad language - fortunately muffled by armpit. This, however, didn't help me get things. Fortunately there was a new gadget to come to the rescue. With this, I can just type my message and it will speak it. Indeed, so efficient is it that as soon as I finish a word, it will say it. (This way I discover my spelling and typing mistakes. Some of these are embarrassing, if not rude - as when I press the adjacent U instead of I in what was meant to be 'bigger', or I instead of U with 'shut'. Unfortunately, with my voice incomprehensible, there's no way out of this.) There is then a long pause while I type the next word, then it says that too. This is a very good patience exercise – also for the person listening to me. (Or the person who *was* listening when the first words came out, but has since walked off.)

Might single words with long pauses sound unnatural? The salesman reassured me: I could pre-programme sentences. "How much of our conversation could we have pre-planned?" I asked. "I don't exactly know," he answered, "but I'll look into it." Would I enjoy such conversations? Or are they for machines to talk to machines?

Pre-programming is, in fact, useful. For the telephone, "I don't speak well. Can I fax you? What is your fax number?" is invaluable. Unfortunately, this is spoken in a voice that *does* speak well, so isn't entirely convincing. Also, it doesn't sound like me, so I have to type a description of who I am, why I've changed my voice and nationality (though Welsh, I now, through the machine, speak with an American accent.) This means a lot of typing, a lot of typing mistakes and, as the screen is too small for so many words, a disjointed sentence. At this point, I invariably discover that no official is allowed to fax me until I've answered several questions in my own voice. (How do they know what it sounds like?)

Pre-programming may have advantages. Teenagers in the house don't. They too like to programme sentences, utilizing what they think is creativity. This means that, on the phone to somebody important, like the bank manager, when I choose 'memory F' (for fax), my machine may speak messages that teenagers think funny. I don't share their humour. Nor, it seems, does my bank manager. Nor do I share their vocabulary. Although I choose the shortest words I can think of to type, most of mine are over four letters - and all require thought. Theirs aren't and don't. It's doubly hard to apologize when, not only is my useless voice barely audible above the mechanically-voiced swearing, but the recipient at the other end has put the phone down. Unfortunately, 'memory F' is my most useful message as it saves non-understood attempted (and failed) telephone conversations. Doubly unfortunately, 'F' is not the only risky letter in the memory programme. Teenagers, it seems, have an extended vocabulary - though not one of my choosing. At times like this, I am glad of the American accent, and hope that my name details weren't still part of the message.

Lesson to be learnt: try harder to keep speech clean.

Further lesson to be learnt: try to anticipate what others will say.

Things nobody dares to sell

Some things, though essential to life, just can't be bought. These you must make. Necessity being the mother of invention, dire necessity has led to some dire inventions.

Amongst the direr was being stuck on the toilet in a friend's house. This stopped being fun when I had read everything three times. I had plenty of time to search for finger holds to pull myself up on. But were there any? Window-sill: too slippery. Plastic deodorizer: too flimsy. Toilet roll holder: too far back. Crack between door and frame: too small. Perhaps I could jam a coin in it and pull on that? But I couldn't hold the coin well enough. A few more attempts and this would get expensive.... There was only one good hold: the door-knob, but frustratingly out of reach. If only it was closer... Or could I lasso it with my belt? This did eventually work. But my success was distinctly qualified. *I* had got up, but my trousers fell down. It did, however, get me thinking: what should I take with me wherever I go?

The solution: nylon cord with a loop at one end, handle at the other. The handle allows a good pull and the loop lets me fix it in several ways to accommodate different size 'anchors' and different distances. Fortunately this device isn't bulky – it's small enough to fit in a pocket. Unfortunately, however, it's uncomfortable to sit on. Nonetheless, I recommend it. (Of course I do; I invented it!)

This gadget does, however, have one disadvantage. It is yet one more item to fill my cargo-trouser pockets or waist-pouch. These are already filled by pocket-survival-kit. This includes (besides wallet, cheque-book, diary and key) mobile phone in case I fall, Rescue Remedy in case I fall badly, notepad and pencil in case I can't speak, penknife in case pencil is blunt, glasses in case I can't see, glasses-case in case I can, so don't need them. The pouch is, therefore, quite heavy. I need to be careful when putting it on, in case it hits me in the

Gadgets and Improvisations

stomach and winds me. Also when taking it off, in case I drop it on my toe. I used to load all this into trousers. The weight being spread, this was safer for toes, but keeping trousers up became an issue.

Elsewhere I have been stuck in bed. Fortunately, my friend had laid in rope for just such a contingency. Attached to the radiator, I could pull myself up. A knotted tail of rope helped me sit from lying, then move along the bed towards the radiator for final lift-off position. As long as I judge the angle of pull correctly, I won't pull the radiator off the wall - or, at least, I haven't yet. This would be a disaster. I would fall. The radiator water would flood the floor and drown me - lying flat as I would be. Worse, the water would be hot, so I would be boiled as well as drowned. Then the heating wouldn't work, so I would be frozen as well as boiled and drowned. Worst of all, as well as being dead, boiled and frozen, my friend wouldn't want me to come to stay again.

So long as nothing like that happens, pulling myself up by the radiator-belayed rope works excellently. But there is one minor snag. The floor is slippery. If I can't position my feet far enough back – and mostly I can't - this means my pull is transferred to a horizontal force on the feet. Consequence: I merely slide off the bed to lie on floor. The problem is socks. Bare feet wouldn't slip. But how could I put on socks when standing? I would need to sit again, put on socks - and then the slip hazard starts all over again....

I do recommend rope, but am less sure about socks. True, they are efficient foot warmers, but, like all efficient things, tend to buy single-function efficiency at the cost of versatility. My friend won't let me nail wooden blocks to the floor, but perhaps if I lay crutches end to end from the far wall... But then, how can I pick the crutches up when standing?

I have also been stuck at table. This was at home - alone. As I pull on the table edge to get myself up, so it slides and wedges my leg between its leg and the built-in seat. This is awkward, and also hurts. Moreover, half standing at table, jammed, is boring after half-an-hour. No alternative but to devise a gadget. This is a plywood 'shoe' on a ply base, jammed back against the seat foot. It works well, but I live in fear of over–zealous visitors 'helping' me by pulling the table out. At best, the leg would jump out of the shoe so I would be trapped next time. At worst, the table would pull off the leg and thereafter hardly be worth sitting at. Also, this would render the shoe unecessary - a waste of effort to have made. I therefore recommend large fluorescent warning signs.

Gadgets and Improvisations

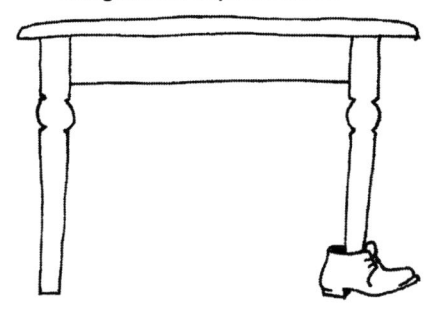

One of my better inventions: could this save the world?

I have also been stuck indoors, able to put on shoes but unable to tie the laces. I could sort-of tie them, but not tight. Moreover, each shoe took fifteen minutes and after that the loose sort-of-tied shoelaces quickly came undone - so add another fifteen minutes ..... The occupational therapist recommended elastic laces, but with only one effective hand, even using a shoehorn, this would make putting on shoes, already hard, worse. So...gadget time.

Anorak draw-strings fasten with spring-loaded toggles, so why not shoes? (True: shoes are at the other end of the body, but toggles don't mind. They even work upside-down.) So easy is this system it gains many admirers – especially as the toggles are bright orange, useful for non-tying shoelaces in the dark. As I invented this, naturally I recommend it. (Also it really does work.) It is important, however, to tuck in the lace ends or I could trip over them if I ran. Fortunately I haven't dreamt about running for about two years. Now I only dream of walking without sticks - so shoelaces are less hazardous than when I was younger.

Another ignominious place to be stuck in is a chair, crutches just out of reach. I can of course lean them against furniture, but then they are free to indulge in crutch behaviour, namely: rotate, slide and fall. Or I can lay them on a table, but then why sit at a table with no space to put anything else on? What I need are crutch clips. Painful as these might sound, they actually make life much safer. Pipe clips make excellent ones. After a little help from a penknife, 22 mm. (3/4") clips are just right for crutches. I have these screwed to my desk and also the wall near the table (the one with the shoe on it's leg.) True: it does make the house look like it's full of half-finished plumbing. But at least my crutches don't fall down.

Another possibility with crutches is to add hooks to the handles. My crutch handles are hollow plastic, closed at the end with a plastic stopper. This makes a useful chamber to store cannabis, semtex, chocolate you don't want children to find, or a mini-survival kit complete with one fish hook, five matches, mini mosquito net (when not catching mini mosquitoes, this doubles a fishing net for mosquito sized fish) and five-climate survival instruction manual. I am working

Gadgets and Improvisations

on a design to add table-gripping hooks without compromising this secret chamber. As this has many potential uses from cripple-bomb to disabled drug-baron, it is clearly more useful than a mere hook.

Lesson to be learnt: Life would be easier if I didn't have to improvise. It might even be easier if I wasn't disabled. But would it be such fun?

Anyway, fun or not-fun, my grandfather taught me that resourcefulness makes everything possible. A surgeon, he made a wooden leg for a turkey and rear-wheels for a dog with paralyzed hindquarters. Both worked well. Unfortunately, I don't have wooden leg skills – neither to make, nor to wear. Rear wheels would be even harder to control – especially on stairs. Anyway, I walk on legs, not on my rear.

5. Everyday Life: Non-everyday problems

Dressing

Days normally start with getting dressed. But dressing isn't simple. Now I have a carer to do it, but until recently I dressed myself. In summer, wearing only a T-shirt and sandals (and the other things, like trousers, necessary for decency), this would take one hour (one and a half with a shower - from which I could only 'air dry': namely not dry myself). Winter with socks, shoes and shirt took longer. By the time I had had breakfast and was ready to start work, it felt like half the day was gone. (Things always feel worse than they are. It was actually only a quarter.)

How can getting dressed take so long? It's quite simple: dressing is complicated. It goes like this: to put on underpants requires a foot through each hole. The first foot is easy: I can flip the underpants over the toe. If I'm lucky, the right foot goes through the right hole. But there are four: right, left, centre and top. Usually - like life - I'm not lucky. Several attempts later and one foot is done, but then the rest of the pants lie on the floor. They must be raised so I can get the other foot in. This requires leaning forward but not falling off the bed. Usually, after several attempts, success: pants over toes. Next, pull pants up. At this stage it becomes clear which hole which foot is in: both in same hole? In separate or wrong holes? Or correct? Each option has a 25 % chance so three-quarters of the time I must start again. This time however I have a 25% chance of doing it right. Well, if not this time, at least *next* time I'll have a 25% chance. Every attempt however increases the risk of my falling off the bed so I must be vigilant. This ensures that I am fully awake.

Next: pulling underpants up. This requires standing. Again, this may sound simple, but takes me several attempts. Now, I am standing, but holding on to the chest of drawers with both hands. Unfortunately, pulling underpants up requires the use of one hand. Like life, I must therefore, let go and trust in fate - or anyway, in balance. So I don't have to bend right down and risk falling on my face, I grip the underpants between my knees. Usually this works, but not always. Sometimes when I stand up, they fall back down around my ankles. If so, I must sit, pull them half up (without falling off the bed) and start again. If, however, they are successfully gripped between the knees, the underpants are in the right place, but won't pull any further up. Choosing the exact moment to ungrip is a precise art - too soon and they fall down, too late and I must pull so hard I risk losing balance. Unfortunately, underpants pulled up on just one side, roll up and jam on the other, so eventually I have to use two hands. Even worse, I have to pull them up behind as well as in front. This is an even greater challenge to balance - requiring even greater trust in destiny. Who would have thought underpants could be so messy to deal with?

Everyday Life: Non-everyday problems

Success at last. Now comes plumbing. This itself is a fiddle. Indeed, to an outside observer it must look as though I am just indecently fiddling. Next I must fix on the leg bag with Velcro straps. These, of course, have fastened onto anything they can find, including each other. Eventually freed, I pass each strap around the leg with one hand (the other is holding the bed edge) While I'm doing this, Velcro - who is strong-willed and mischievous - is searching out a new target: sock, sock on other leg, laces on nearby shoe, even my shirtsleeve. Despite such interference, I eventually manage to wind the strap around my leg. But when I reach for the Velcro end, the released strap unwinds. This can take so many attempts I'm tempted to let go of the bed and risk falling off. Anything for an easy pee! Or I could just not fasten the Velcro? Having tried the brick-on-willy thing once, this, however, is not an option.

Now trousers. Anything difficult with underpants is even harder with trousers. As my legs like to draw towards each other, the right leg wants to go down the left leg-hole. I usually stop it. Often, however, I only half-stop it, so the big toe goes one way, the other toes the other. This means my foot jams in the trouser crotch. It can jam quite tight, so removing trousers from toes takes a little while. Eventually, however, I have two legs in separate leg-holes, hopefully the right ones, the right way round. (Even professional carers can make mistakes here. One, used only to dressing women, likes to put the trouser zip at the back. For men, this can bring problems.) Eventually, even I can complete this stage, but not without much time taken in the process.

Lesson to be learnt: a foot in the crotch slows everything down.

Eventually both feet are in separate trouser-legs. But I can't pull one side of the trousers up when my other foot pins the other trouser-leg to the floor. Even once this is sorted out, I can't stand up in them until both trouser-legs are pulled up past the heel. At this point, my toes like to jam in the hem. This breaks the stitching, so enlarging this toe trap for the morrow. Trousers unfortunately, have two legs, so problems with the first leg must be repeated with the second.

Finally I'm ready to stand and pull them up. But as my trousers are heavy with pocket contents they want to fall about my ankles. As I'm slow, they are more ready than I am to do their thing before I can do mine. Usually it's not too hard to get them half-way up, then the belt catches on the bed-frame behind me and down they go again. I could of course step away from the bed, but then I tread on the trousers. How to get them out from under my feet without losing balance? This would mean another step away from the bed, but I'm not keen on that. As long as I'm close enough to fall back on it, I'm more or less safe.

Next, I must sit and put on a T-shirt. This is relatively easy. Now, I can lie back to zip up my trousers, struggle with the button and fasten my belt. Pulling myself back to sitting up is less easy, but so far I've always managed it. (Obviously! How could I write this book lying on my back?)

Now comes sandal-putting-on-time. Again, left sandal is easy to put on, but it does require a dangerous lean to fasten it. Right sandal isn't. It needs one hand to raise my foot and one to put on sandal – so doubling falling-off-bed risk. Likewise it needs two hands - and, as far as balance goes, trust in destiny - to fasten the buckle. My watch strap could well take another ten minutes, but it never does. If I haven't succeeded in five, the watch goes in my pocket. (Also it's less dangerous. One of the very few low-risk bits of life.) Eventually I'm totally dressed, more or less (on the surface) respectable and everything (except remembering how my legs work) is sorted. But one hour gone.

Lesson to be learnt: getting up (and dressed) is good for the will.

Half a day to get dressed can feel frustratingly long. From my hitch-hiking days (sometimes waiting eight hours for a lift), I should have learnt that everything will work out right in the end. Just as I learnt to enjoy walking empty roads amidst beautiful mountains, I should have enjoyed the challenges of dressing. After all, it was never half a day wasted, but quarter of a day of will-exercise.

Nowadays I have a carer to dress and undress me. Initially, I resisted this. I didn't want a different stranger everyday to whiz in, whiz me into bed (in this case, a slow motion whiz) in the early evening, whiz me out, mid-morning, and whiz off. This would make me feel like a sack of potatoes. Yes, it's true: I do walk almost as fast as one - but I don't like to be treated like one. In the event, however, I found the carers all really cared, did much more than they were contracted for, and - far from being whizzing strangers - have all become my friends.

Occasionally, however, carers change. This means I have to tell the new one about everything I need done, *how* to do it, where everything is, and in what efficient order to do it. Unfortunately, I can't. Until they know me, they can't understand my voice. This can be frustrating. With one new carer, I had to resort to written instructions. At least, that was my intention. I made signs for a pencil and paper. She then started to seat me on the toilet. This led me to wonder how she normally treated patients. True: paper does have something to do with using the toilet. But a pencil?

Lesson to be learnt: misunderstandings can be dangerous. They can even hurt.

Dressing-by-carer goes much quicker, but even here, things can go less than perfectly. Carers often do unnecessary things, like washing my back. I *know* this is clean; I've *never* seen any dirt there. Even they can do things wrong, from mis-buttoning shirts (but fortunately, most have spare buttonholes) to fastening my leg-bag's Velcro strap to my sock. Result: I tread on both bag and sock - not only squelchingly embarrassing, but I also get a cold leg. I never remember healthy-days showering and dressing being funny but doing things wrong adds humour. Unfortunately, if we laugh too much, even professional carers can forget important things. Hence, I occasionally have to remind them that it is more discreet to wear my pee-bag inside my trousers instead of connecting it after they're pulled up. Or, after putting on my shoes, that I usually wear trousers to breakfast. Or, when being put in bed, that I indulge in that odd Welsh custom of not wearing shoes in bed. I'm glad I'm not the only one who ever does things wrong!

Lesson to be learnt: not all habits are bad.

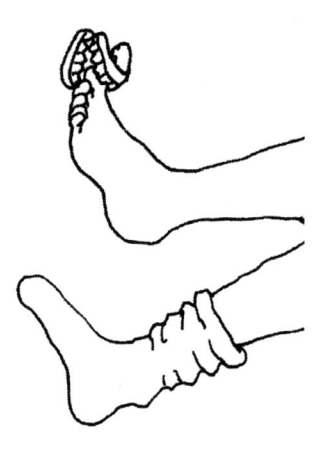

If my foot is touched the wrong way, my leg can suddenly spasm. This can make dressing-by-carer painful.

Eating

I love good food but not all food loves me. Also the technicalities of eating make mealtimes difficult. Apart from choking, my tongue won't move things around, so I can only chew in the front of my mouth. Anything too large needs, therefore, to be only half in or my mouth gets jammed, the teeth just ineffectually sliding past the stationary lump in the centre. Chewing food half in, half out of, my mouth means I dribble. Try as I (sometimes) do, I am nonetheless a messy eater. Dribble, slobber, choking and power-jet regurgitation don't endear me to dinner table neighbours.

Survival technique: dress for dinner with draped towels - just as for a haircut, which, though it doesn't taste as good, is no messier. This keeps me clean but doesn't inspire confidence in others.

I can't eat hard things, like apple cubes, that jam in the throat. Nor dry grains, like whole-meal husks, that stick in it. Nor fibres or strings like tomato-skins that leave half in the mouth while the other half is swallowed. Although I try to explain this, cooks often just describe me as a "no-nuts person". Fortunately, being a father, I know this isn't true. I also like nuts. Unfortunately, the nicest and most nutritious food can be the hardest to eat. Instant speed-food sludge is effortless, but doesn't do me much good. Is this a lesson for life? Things worth doing, nourishing relationships and personal growth are never difficulty-free. Easy ones are ...easy - but bring no benefit.

Eating difficulties have, however, given me an idea for my next invention: electric false-teeth. Ideally, these would be three-speed; also battery-powered, as wires dribbling from the mouth might look odd. The remote-controller should be sized to discretely fit in a pocket – but you must be careful not to knock it, lest the teeth start up.

One aspect of my illness is that muscles like to contract. They will do this on their own, without my telling them to do so. One result is involuntary teeth clenching. If this happens when eating, I bite the spoon. Normally, this only means a jolt to my jaw (and what little remains of my brain) and a loud clang. There is a risk, however, that spoon and contents will fly out of my mouth across the table. Unfortunately, I know very few people who enjoy being fed this way.

Another problem is that when I think of speaking, something must shift in my throat so I choke. Hence when someone asks me a question and my mouth is full I must either turn rudely away or risk choking over their plate, lap or face. I'm sure I could improve with practice, but few people ask me to dinner these days.

Lesson to be learnt: food is only nice once. Sharing food isn't popular.

Drinking

Drinking presents three difficulties: obtaining drink, lifting cup and swallowing. To obtain drink, my electronic gadget is handy. I just type the words in and an American voice says "I...want...T." Initially my family were affronted when an invisible stranger had apparently walked into the house and demanded a drink. Now they just ignore him.

Next comes cup-raising. This is normally easy but, as even my better arm tends to flop without warning, can be disastrous with a pint of hot tea. Doubly disastrous as, apart from leaving an embarrassingly positioned stain, this is a bad place to be boiled. Indeed, trebly disastrous as it's a large-scale waste of tea. I therefore use two hands. In France, coffee is traditionally drunk from a bowl. With elbows on the table to increase stability and two hands holding bowl, this brings my face over steaming coffee. Aromatic and delightful – until I attempt to drink. This causes my nose to submerge. As long as I don't drown or scald nose, this is funny – anyway for anyone else. But laughing is not the most stable way to hold a bowl of liquid. This slops from front to back and – worse - from back to front.

Lesson to be learnt: buy dark trousers. (They're also better for travelling. I learnt this holding a cup of brown coffee between my white-trousered thighs when the car went over a bump.)

Additional lesson to be learnt: Whether lecturing, travelling, practicing incontinence or anywhere in France, don't wear white trousers. What these things have in common isn't clear. But clearly - as in life - relationships aren't simple.

Alternatively I could give up coffee. Most experts and all food-faddists agree that water is healthier. I'm sure they are right, but nowadays water is hard for me to drink. It is the thinnest of (non-alcoholic) liquids. Moreover it is usually drunk cold which slows down my throat muscles. This combination makes water easy to choke on, especially when I'm tired. Choking means first a sudden face-level jet-spray over whoever is near me, then horrific grating noises as I gasp for breath. At this point the wet person is supposed to want to help me.

But technology to the rescue! Fortunately, modern science has invented a powder that turns water into a flavourless porridge. Unfortunately, the researchers would have done better to patent this as a cement-substitute. As it thickens slowly, it's tempting to put too much in, so turning water into thick goo (or glue) ten minutes later. Personally I don't find flavourless goo appealing to drink. I prefer tea, which, being hot, and slightly thicker than water I still (fortunately) can drink without choking. Isn't there a Transylvanian proverb about something being thicker than water?

Alcohol is a different matter. Spirits evaporate in the mouth so cause me to choke instantly - even before I swallow them. This isn't fair: I'm drunk before I have drunk anything. Less strong drink is easier to swallow but affects my legs within seconds. After even a tiny drink I can't walk straight or speak without slur. I can't even do those without drinking – but at least I could then honestly wear the "I'm not drunk. I have MS/Stroke/MND/ALS" (delete as appropriate) T-shirt. This also isn't fair: I act as though I'm drunk without the chance to drink anything.

Breathing

Most people don't think about breathing. I do, anyway at night. More precisely, my body makes me think about how to start breathing again when it stops. Despite never having learnt this in school, I'm told this is important. Breathing is said to make life easier. (Did I learn anything useful in school?) I just don't always know *how* to start breathing again! (Unfortunately, school didn't teach me this either.)

When I go to sleep, what feels like a flap in my throat, nose or airway closes with a clunk - exactly like a vacuum-cleaner nozzle suddenly suffocating on a piece of paper. This usually wakes me up (I assume it *always* does or I wouldn't be writing this book). Shifting head and neck position clears this, presumably letting the hinged flap flop open. Unfortunately, this can't be fully tested till I go back to sleep and my muscles relax again. This can happen many times a night. Stopping breathing may sound frightening, but actually isn't. I know I probably will breathe again - that's as much as any of us knows. It is, however, quite tiring and definitely tiresome. Cranial osteopathy helped greatly, and with careful body positioning, I now can sleep through most nights - but for waking to turn over. By day, this never more than half happens. This means I never less than half-breathe and occasionally make strange stentorian snorts. This may be good for drawing attention in a crowd, but I don't always want attention. Sometimes, I would just prefer to breathe.

Anti-clunk head-positioning gets me breathing again. Unfortunately, however, breath problems aren't over. If I get the position wrong, every breath snorts gratingly. This keeps me - and probably everyone else in the house - awake. Snort-control - interspersed with more clunk-control, if I move into the wrong position - can take many posture adjustments till it works both asleep and awake. None of this helps uninterrupted sleep.

Lesson to be learnt: don't take anything, even our daily breath, for granted.

Further lesson to be learnt: illness raises consciousness. Who else ever thinks about how to breathe?

Sleeping

Combining building, vegetable growing, architecture and single parenting, I used to sleep soundly and go to sleep within seconds (probably fifteen) of my head hitting the pillow. Not now. Nowadays I do no physical work, and mental work has never been known to encourage deep sleep.

Going to sleep is rarely a problem, but after a while my hips ache. One way to avoid this is to sleep with a pillow between my knees. Unfortunately, it doesn't like to stay there. Soon Pillow and I are fighting for bedspace. I only tried this once - the pillow won. The other way is to roll over. This is simple, non-adversarial - but a major operation. After much stretching, I can usually reach the side of the bed to pull on. Thereafter rolling, though hard, is now possible. I must also be careful not to fall out. As I roll, the bedclothes roll with me, but they are less careful than me and keep on going towards the floor. Once I am safe these have to be grabbed and hauled back on the bed. Naturally they no longer want to cover my feet. As they are, by now, diagonal to the bed, I walk my hands along the quilt edge till I find a corner and pull it into alignment. Much wriggling and ineffectual foot movements and I can now find out whether the quilt is along or across the bed. If across, I give up on the quilt and try to shape my body to fit under it - again being careful not to fall out, and to keep my head and neck optimally positioned for breathing. By now, of course, I am thoroughly awake.

Everyday Life: Non-everyday problems

Before I can get back to sleep, small thoughts creep into my brain. These are followed by bigger ones. These in turn by worries about all the things that urgently need doing but that I can no longer do and my defective (indeed thoroughly dud) voice won't let me phone someone else to do. By now I am thoroughly not going to sleep.

The first thing to do with night thoughts is to roll over. This way all the thoughts that have collected on one side of the brain have to trickle through to the other. On their way many get lost. This really does work, but in my case rolling over is a major process. Indeed it's what thoroughly woke me up in the first place. The next thing to do is to lie in the recovery position. This also works, but to get there usually loses my bedclothes. As sleeping without bedclothes won't be sleeping, I usually therefore get into a half recovery position with half my bedclothes and only go half to sleep.

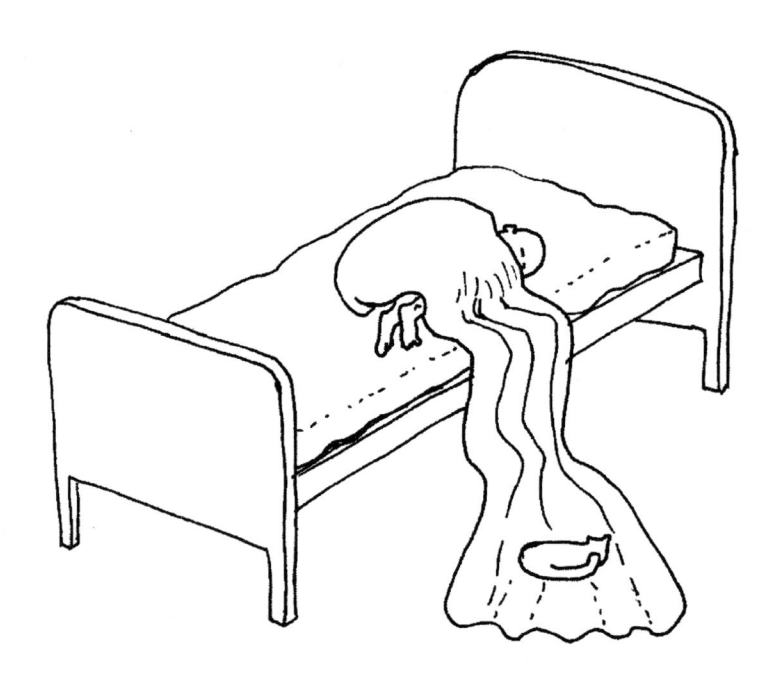

It's easier to sleep if fully adjusted to your situation.

Next I try to remember my day backwards. Starting with where I now am (half in bed), I try to remember the events that preceded this, then those that preceded those and so on, finishing with waking in the morning. This takes great concentration as my mind keeps wandering. The more it wanders, the more naughty thoughts creep in and take over. The more I can concentrate, the more tired I get so the harder it is to complete the whole days review; I'm usually asleep before I have even got back to teatime. Unfortunately I'm often too tired to concentrate and so take the lazy course, letting the Naughty Thought Gang creep back in.

Fortunately I have one last technique – the best, and also one easy to repeat. I recite a verse, meditation or prayer slowly. One or, at most two, words per slow, measured breath. By the end, my mind is calmed and my thoughts have gone back to sleep. I use the 'Lord's Prayer'. Is it sacrilege to 'use' it like this? Both prayer and day review are about more important things than going to sleep. The slow prayer allows me to concentrate on, and live into the meaning of every word. The day review helps me recognize the soul significance of every event, how it affected me. Also it helps me see life - or anyway, one day of life - no longer as a chaos of random events to which I am victim, but as a chain of consequences, causes and linkages for which my (albeit thoughtless) actions are responsible. Like history read backwards (technically demanding as few books are written backwards), this makes it easier both to understand *and* to go to sleep. It also feels like washing and fortifying the soul. What better state to carry into sleep? No wonder it prepares me to sleep.

It may seem odd that inner-development exercises are such good somnumbulizers, but perhaps there is a reason. After all, it's usual in life, that the ethically right course invariably turns out to be the most sustainably practical, whereas the amoral pragmatic one doesn't endure. Who would have thought sustainability would prove to be a spiritual, not material-value, issue? Who would have thought this had anything to do with sleep?

Lesson to be learnt: the wrong thing done for the right reason is right; the right thing done for the wrong reason is wrong; but the really, really right thing transforms the reason. But what is the 'right' reason? Right for me is often wrong for someone else. And anyway, what is the reason? There are usually many layers: right, wrong, don't know, not aware of.... And anyway (again), whatever our actions, right or wrong, they've led to life as it is now. As life isn't wrong, they can't have been wrong. Or...

More important lesson to be learnt: ethics is complicated, too complicated when I'm tired. It would be simpler just to go to sleep!

6. Falls

When I say my condition is painless, this is not entirely true about falls. Though some are comical, all falls are discouraging. Fortunately, most have no lasting effect. Some, however, cause permanent injury. Some even hurt.

You name it and I've fallen in it or on it: concrete, grass, puddle, bath; wooden slatting, steel cattle-grid, soft heather, prickly gorse; flower bed, soft bed, off bed; into chair, out of chair; street pavement, railway platform, railway train, airport. I've fallen up stairs, down stairs and on the level. I've landed in dog shit, sheep shit, mud, water, face into compost bucket – a disaster: split bucket, wasted compost. I've fallen over cat, dog, slug; slipped on water, slime, fluff, grease. I've had my crutch tripped over, kicked away, blown away, even taken away by someone trying to help. (Help is always more effective, if aided by brains.) I've broken nose, rib, hurt spine, knocked myself out, been temporarily 100% paralyzed. Based on experience, I have now decided I don't like falling.

I used to land softly but fall often – at the worst stage, three in one day; seventeen a month. Most didn't hurt, and I could get up easily. While each was a blow to morale, I could rejoice in the tally as it was necessary evidence to convince the government that I was disabled. (I wonder, however, are there less dramatic ways of convincing governments?) Nowadays I fall less frequently, but land hard and can't get up. Of course, I do try *not* to fall. I also try to get up. I'm not sure, however, whether either makes any difference.

A typical fall starts with the realization that I'm out of balance. My reactions are too slow to counter this so, with slow motion inevitability, the fall starts. Fortunately, I have time to look around and choose the best, or least worst, place to land. Usually I can trust my body enough to hit this target. Unfortunately, falls on the back don't give this luxury. Falls to the front I try to absorb by landing on outstretched arms. The left one, however, collapses immediately, leaving my face to cushion the final impact. Still, at least with a slow motion fall I knew what I was going to hit - even if this would have to be nose first!

All this has helped teach me the Zen art of acceptance. Prior to being ill, my only experience of Zen was eating at a chip-shop whose neon sign proclaimed FRO**ZEN FOODS**. Now, life (or dying) ensures I practice it every day.

Lesson to be learnt: accept the inevitable; but not falling at all is better.

Unfortunately, falls often *are* nose first. This is not good for noses - they aren't designed for falling on. In fact, I broke one (my only one). I didn't know I'd broken it as, though it hurt, I didn't think it hurt *enough* to qualify. But it bled. I didn't know noses could bleed so much – much more than a spilt pint of milk - and you can't (or anyway, I didn't want to) call the dog to lick it up. Bleeding like that made me feel heroic. Nonetheless, I found the appeal of feeling heroic had suddenly sharply diminished. Seeing all that blood is not good for morale, so, if anybody wants to try this at home, I would recommend switching the light off first.

After five days – when I dared touch my nose to wipe away snot – I noticed it clicked. I was persuaded to go to the doctor. He made an appointment with the squashed-nose specialist. By the time I saw him it was fourteen days after nose-smash. The squashed-nose-ist was not impressed. Yes, it was broken, but not flat enough for someone as highly qualified as him. He did, however, offer to break it again. I declined the offer.

Breaking my rib also didn't hurt much. This was a self-inflicted injury - not the ground's fault. That was far too soft to hurt but a cold wind had made my fist involuntarily clench. It was this I landed on. When I shouted to my daughter some fifty metres away only a whisper came out. I had to whisper for about ten minutes till she didn't hear me, but came back to the spot where I now wasn't standing. My inability to speak above a whisper did seem a bit odd, but I didn't think anything was amiss. The children and dog appreciated this - it meant they never heard commands they didn't want to hear. So rib-breaking has some advantages. (Indeed, from my dog I should have learnt that selective hearing lets you do whatever you want. Wouldn't life be easier for everyone if everyone could do whatever they wanted? Of course! But also it would be harder for everyone else. Who should have priority: everyone? Or everyone else? Or just deaf dogs?)

Two days later, however, I began to wonder about the bowl-shaped hollow in my ribs, so went to the doctor. She sent me straight to hospital for an X-ray. There, I was immediately put in a wheelchair (I'd been walking for two days) wheeled ten metres to a casualty couch, had a huge needle inserted in my arm and waited for an X-ray. A junior doctor came in and wanted to connect pain-killer drip to the needle. I said I preferred to know when I was doing something wrong, not be numbed. Anyway it didn't hurt too badly. After an hour, a more senior doctor appeared and asked me the cure for broken ribs. Somewhat surprised that he didn't know, I said I thought no bandages, splints or slings - just time. "Right" he said, "So there's no point in having an X-ray." (So what was the point in going to hospital?).

The rib hurt for three months, but not too badly. In fact it only hurt when I was doing something - like breathing. Some movements, particularly getting out of bed, were quite unpleasant, almost enough to put me off getting up. This was the best excuse I've ever had to stay in bed all day. With sufficient gritting of teeth, getting up was just manageable - but not sneezing! Not only is it hard to grit teeth and sneeze at the same time, but I would feel a sneeze coming and think "Oh no! This is going to *really* hurt!" The sneeze would build up with a breath intake – then, at the one point you can *never* stop a sneeze, stop. My body saved me. Thank you dear body. This did, however, put me off sneezing.

Falls

In any case, sneezes aren't good for falls. (They may be good for falls, but not for me, as I'm actually trying to *avoid* falls.) When I sneeze, my whole body jerks, so whenever I feel one coming, I look round for something to hold onto or I will surely fall. But sometimes there's nothing – no door-frame, counter or table: I'm in the middle of the room. The sneeze builds up.... and stops! It seems my body looks after me. Thank you again, dear body. You are a good friend. In fact, uncooperative though you mostly are, I can't easily do without you.

I should have learnt not to worry. Indeed, I should have learnt this from my mother. She used to say: "Don't worry. It may never happen!" As a child, I never found this very encouraging. My own (adult) version is: "What's the worst that could happen?" (Presumably: death.) Put together, this makes: "Don't worry. I (or you) may never die more than once." This is meant to be reassuring – but not everyone finds it so. Or might it be better to expect to die (and therefore to live) *more* than once?

I didn't even die after my most serious fall. This occurred in a friend's bathroom. My socks slipped on the plastic floor and I pivoted past my handholds, hitting the back of my head on the basin. And then I was staring at a view I had never seen before. Nor could I understand where I was or why I was looking at this mystifying view. Eventually I worked out that it was water beads on the shower screen. I couldn't look around; my eyes wouldn't move. I tried to shout – but nothing. I'm not even sure whether or how I could breathe. There was nothing frightening about this, but it did seem a little odd. It eventually dawned on me that I must have fallen. Fortunately I wasn't dead (or, at least, I thought I wasn't). Fortunately also, nothing hurt, but complete inability to move didn't seem quite normal. Clearly things weren't ideal.

My friends had heard me fall and arrived about a minute later. They eased me to a more comfortable position. But it wasn't comfortable! My back hurt - not badly, but not nice. I tried to move to relieve it – and started to writhe. My friends looked terrified so I told them I wasn't in pain; at least I *tried* to tell them. What actually came out was an awful groaning. The more I tried to reassure them that I was 'alright' the more I groaned and the more alarmed they looked.

One got a bottle of Bach Flower 'Rescue Remedy' and poured a few drops onto my tongue. Instantly I could speak! (It may not have been instantaneous; perhaps it took half a second, definitely less than one second). I told them I was alright (meaning I wasn't dead) but looking back on it, I clearly wasn't. But also, I clearly wasn't dead - even they could have seen that! At the time, I was relieved not to be dead so not at all worried. Had I been dead I probably wouldn't have been worried either.

There is a theory that the bliss reported by people who die (but don't stay dead) is just the brain closing down. My own experience of closed-down brain was anything but blissful. Dying-for-real has got to be better than falling in bathrooms.

To avoid wasting a day or two in hospital, I got my friends to check for concussion by shining a torch in my eyes to see if my pupils reacted. This was the third time I had needed such a test and each time I passed. Unfortunately I've since discovered this is only a small part of the test – hence easy to pass. Afterwards though, the memory scared me. Also I had two weeks headache, felt rotten, didn't enjoy giving a lecture the next day and worried I may have cracked my skull. I therefore do not recommend falling in bathrooms.

Lesson to be learnt: groaning and writhing don't necessarily mean agony.

Additional lesson to be learnt: everyone after an accident says "I'm alright" - but they probably aren't. What they actually mean is "I'm not dead" – which is anyway obvious, so why do they bother to say it?

Precautionary lesson to be learnt: in bathrooms, wear crampons (or carry an ice-axe).

My most painful fall wasn't hard. In fact it was really two half-falls. In the first half descent, I hit my back on the edge of an antique table. The second was, therefore, slower. Once safely on the floor, I was relieved to discover that I could move. Evidently my back wasn't broken - and fortunately, nor was the table - but I didn't really feel like getting up, so spent the afternoon under a blanket, my head on a pillow, in the middle of the floor. The table looked down at me, no hint of sympathy in the expression on its bottom. Although much older than me, it seems it's also much tougher. I had a visible bruise – and my spine hurt - for eight months. Table seemed unscathed.

Lesson to be learnt: don't pick a fight with anything older than yourself. It has had many more years to learn survival skills.

The most demoralizing falls don't necessarily hurt. In the first, my stick slipped on wet paving. I wasn't injured, but it felt like everything I had relied on couldn't be trusted. With crutches, I did the same thing again on wet concrete. This time, only one crutch slipped, so I slowly pivoted, fell on my back and hit my head on bricks edging a flower-bed. True: this wasn't entirely painless but (apparently) it also wasn't fatal. After these experiences, I now don't enjoy rain. They also taught me that I couldn't rely on anything – not sticks, not crutches, not even rough concrete. Concrete, in fact, is the most treacherous of surfaces. It looks high-friction anti-slip, but grows slippery, invisible moulds.

Lesson to be learnt: in slippery situations, don't rely on the usual props.

Other falls have had more comic outcomes. Twice I've ended up on my back, fortunately unhurt. But unfortunately I was unable to make myself heard. Fortunately again, both times I had a mobile phone in my pocket. Unfortunately, although it was only to the next room that I needed to phone, both times there were long romantic teenage telephone conversations going on. This, therefore, meant long waits – the first, lying on wet concrete in the rain; the second on a draughty, cold tile floor - but at least I could lie comfortably. The third time I did this, however, nobody answered, only the answerphone saying I was out - which wasn't at all true. I was in, but on the floor. In the end, after much wriggling and failing to get up, I gave up trying and pressed my alarm-button. Although worn around my neck for easy access, my many layers of winter clothes meant I had to half-undress to find which layers it was hiding between. The response was rapid. Within five minutes I heard voices. By good fortune, friends had come to visit. They got me up and then rang the emergency service to cancel the ambulance, now on its way. But here the problems started. The voice at the other end said "Hello, Mr. Day. Can you hear me?" My friend - female, so obviously not Mr. Day - answered "Hello. Can you hear me?" Repeat of "Hello, Mr. Day. Can you hear me?" My friend repeated "Hello. Can you hear me?" There were about five such exchanges until Other-End-Voice said "I can hear you. What is the matter?" Friend then told Other-End-Voice that I was unhurt and didn't need an ambulance. Other-End-Voice was quite annoyed and said it couldn't be cancelled. Moreover, I wasn't allowed to eat or drink anything and would have to go to hospital for a check-up. I therefore quickly drank my tea before I heard this. (Remember: I am slow, so this time, I must have heard slowly.) About twenty minutes later, the ambulance crew arrived - very nice people, despite their over-controlling controller. Within minutes, my daughter and friend rushed in, then next-door neighbours. Calling an ambulance seems a good way to have a party. Unfortunately, although I wasn't hurt, I wasn't quite in party mood either, although it certainly was good for a laugh. This episode did, however give me an idea for my next invention: an inflatable ambulance as a cure for loneliness.

Lesson to be learnt: there is nothing like a tragedy for getting friends to come round.

Additional lesson: be careful of pushing buttons.

In yet another greasy-concrete fall, I fortunately was with a friend. She grabbed my arm, but not in time to save me. It did mean, however, that I fell slowly and didn't hurt myself. But how to get up? My feet slipped on the greasy concrete, and she wasn't strong enough to lift me. To get me half-way up, she fetched a low stool and managed to get this under my chest. This was much better. I was no longer lying in a puddle, so part of me was no longer getting wetter. (It couldn't.) As it was raining, however, the other part was. My friend considerately fetched an umbrella. Even better, I was now out of the rain. But I still couldn't get up. Umbrellas are actually no help here. All I could do was wriggle like an ineffectual fish. This also was no help. Fish don't stand so don't know how to get up. Nor, with my trunk supported and limbs free to make fishy movements, did I. Unfortunately, this was so comic I started

Falls

to laugh. So did she. Unfortunate because, when laughing, it's hard to look pathetic enough to need rescue. Fortunately, we heard a tractor on the road and she went to stop it and summon help. Fortunately again, tractors are loud enough to drown the sound of laughter, so good rescue vehicles. Well equipped with front-end-loader, link-box and winch, this seemed perfect for the task. In the event, however, we didn't need the tractor to get me up; the driver proved sufficient.

Lesson to be learnt: there is more to life than keeping dry.

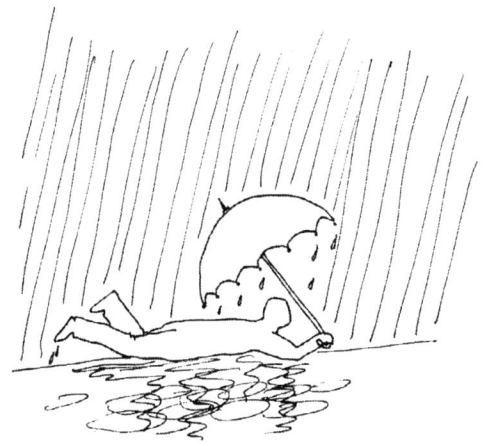

After falling, it's always better to keep dry.

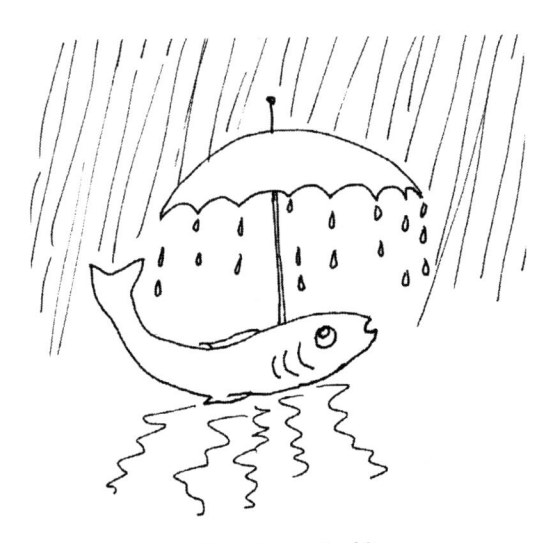

How it actually felt.

One good thing about falling (there must be one!) is that I can rejoice in every day that I don't; other people get despondent about getting older. This is like rain. Every day it rains, I'm glad that I won't need to regret working indoors.

Every day it doesn't, I'm even gladder that it's fine! Another good thing is that it has taught me to count.

An even better thing is that strangers rush to help. True: most don't know how. But good intent far outweighs any incompetence – spirit-lifting for me and heart-rewarding for them. It seems my illness is a key to human warmth that many don't dare open in other situations – so something to be grateful for. I learnt also that how people *are*, deep – and usually concealed – within themselves, is more important than any knowledge or skills they may – but usually don't - have. All this is about compassion: love. Love from so many, unexpected, people gives hope. Hope in a world, which outwardly doesn't offer so much.

Falls - and my inability to stop them - have taught me a lot about learning to accept life. But I'm still not as accepting as was my father. All through World War II in Burma, with friends killed and himself wounded, he regularly prayed "Dear God, thank you for everything." I wish I had got that far - but I'm less keen on going to Burma. It's not a good idea to go somewhere that keeps changing its name – I may never find it. And it's an even less good idea to go to war. When will world leaders realize that going to war does nothing to stop them falling?

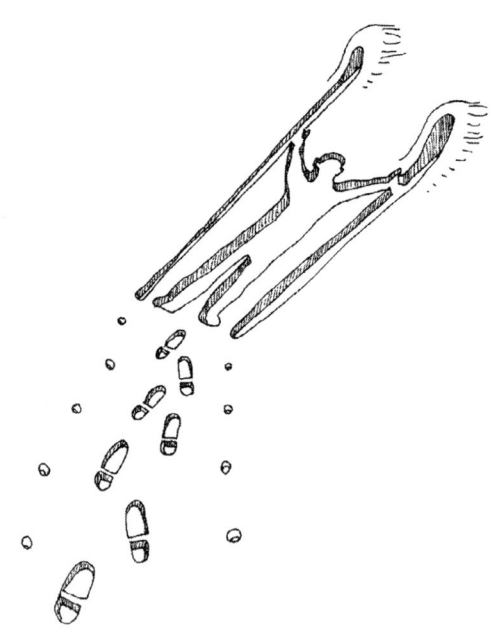

Disabled tracking is easy in snow.

At Home and Elsewhere

7. Beds I have known

When it's hard to get into, out of, or turn over in bed, beds become significant. I now have quite a close relationship to mine. Not exactly a loving relationship, but we do sleep together regularly.

My previous bed was aging. This didn't affect its looks, but did its performance. Also, it was becoming soft. This made it hard to get out of. Moreover, its soft edge twice tipped me onto the floor. Once was when reaching for a dressing-gown - the sneaky edge let me down so I overbalanced. On another occasion, coughing bounced me out. I tried to climb up the bed, but my feet kept slipping on the wooden floorboards. Fortunately, as my mobile phone doesn't work in the bedroom and my voice is weak, I carry a whistle for safety back-up. At night, this is always within reach - from the bed. Unfortunately however, from the floor, it was *out* of reach. (That wasn't really important as my lungs are so weak that when I blow the whistle, it makes a faint dribbling sound, barely audible even in the next room.) Between no whistle and no voice, it took most of an hour till I could make myself heard and get rescued. In winter, it's cold on the floor, but I did manage to pull the bed-clothes down to keep me company. Nonetheless, floor is not my favourite bed.

Lesson to be learnt: When you can't go any lower, remember that warmth is all around you – just waiting to be reached.

When the district nurse offered to arrange a motorized adjustable bed, it seemed a good idea. It did, of course, take about eight months to come. This felt a long time but, for the government, was fairly quick. When it did eventually arrive, however, I wasn't so sure it *was* a good idea!

First, I got a letter informing me of the delivery date and requiring me to remove my own bed by 8 a.m. Not easy when disabled. Nor was it so easy to arrange someone to move this bed at 7:30 as this is right in the middle of the "Hurry, I'm late for the school bus." rush. As I'm so slow dressing, I would have to get up around six if I was to be ready in time to lose my bed and not go with it. I wondered what would happen if there were delays or the delivery-men couldn't find the house. (Where I live, most things only arrive one or two days *after* their notified delivery date!) Arranging - at short notice - a team to put the bed *back* wouldn't be easy. Arranging a repeat early-morning team to take it away again, would quickly start to use up friends.

All (anyway most) worries in vain. Two men arrived with the bed bits. Many journeys through the house with more bits. Clearly, my bed would be an impressive assembly. I stood in the doorway and watched the bed grow.

Beds I have known

It was HUGE - about eighteen inches longer than its predecessor - as befits a More Important Bed. But 7' 10" is big in a small room. Also, with its side fences, it was quite a bit wider. And it was higher, with sides and head and foot boards making it higher again. Above all this stood a steel 'monkey pole'.

The men proudly turned to me to demonstrate how it worked and give me safety warnings. First the controls: the fitter showed me how the bed folded, tilted and rose. I must be careful, he warned, not to go too high or the monkey pole would go through the ceiling, so powerful was the motor. I realized it would therefore go through the roof as well! He demonstrated. The bed and pole approached the ceiling - but the man was looking at me to see if I understood how careful I must be. I foresaw imminent calamity, but my speech and movements are slow. As hurriedly as I was slowly able, I stopped him and begged him to take the monkey pole off. But wouldn't I need it? I assured him I wouldn't. Whether or not I *did* need it, I didn't know - but even less did I need a hole in the roof! Somewhat grudgingly, after all the work of fitting it, he removed the pole and leant it against the wall. It now took up most of the remaining space in the little room. He then told me the bed couldn't be pushed into the corner or, if I pressed the tip command, it would demolish the wall, so strong - and strong-willed - was the motor. It seemed I was doomed to a huge, monstrously ugly, malevolently powerful bed in the middle of the room.

Suitably located away from all walls, he put the wheel-brakes on, warning me not to do this with bare feet - unless I didn't mind it biting a bit off my foot. I did (mind) - so determined never to! Next, I climbed onto the bed to try it out. I raised the side fences. They clicked reassuringly into place. After lying a moment, I tried to lower the fences. They wouldn't. At this point, I discovered that - for safety reasons - they could only be lowered by somebody *outside* the bed. (This is because disabled people can't be trusted - everyone knows cripples are a bit ga-ga.) Just as well I learnt this now, while the fitters were still there! I silently vowed never to use the fences - and hoped no uninitiated well-meaning friend would ever shut me in - potentially for life.

As a parting shot, one of the men warned me not to let any dogs or cats go under the bed, lest they become dog (or cat) sandwich should I lower it. Unfortunately my cat isn't good at remembering commands and instructions given the previous day, let alone remembering them all year.

I thought it wise to practice controlling the bed, but quickly learnt that if I asked it to do two things at once it would just groan and give up. It obviously had strictly limited intelligence. Should I drop the controls, however, Bed has me in its absolute power. Clearly, with this combination of power and intelligence, it is World Leader class.

Beds I have known

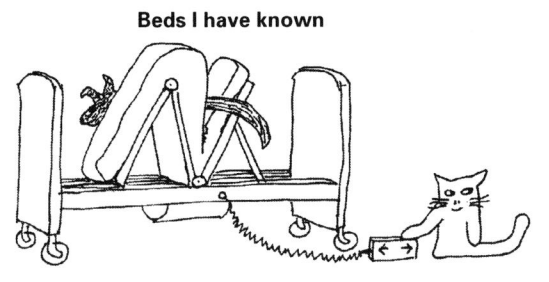

Dog sandwich.

By now, I was thoroughly wary of the bed. It didn't feel like a friend at all! Nonetheless, with the old bed gone, I had no choice but to sleep in it. That night, I decided to try out its abilities and see what advantages I could find. After pressing a few wrong buttons - which raised it quite high - I found the head-raising button. Having come so high, I thought I ought to check how far it would go, before children discovered they could play with it. High! It rose to about five feet above the floor. At its lowest point, the room is only six feet high, so, with mattress thickness and nose length, this meant my nose was about two inches below the ceiling. Fortunately I hadn't operated tilt or sandwich commands, nor raised the head too much, or I wouldn't have been looking at the ceiling, but at the sky.

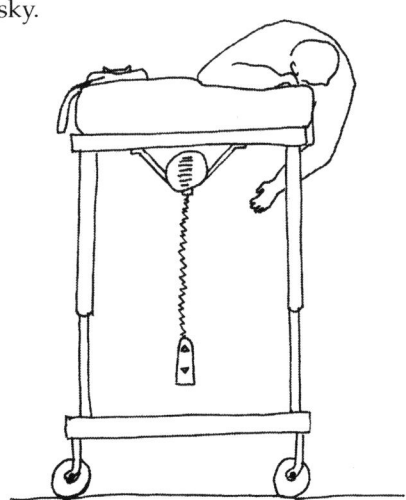

Dropped controls mean losing control.

This height gave a good view: one I'd never had in bed before. There was, however, one disadvantage: the bed was far too high to get out of - but no matter. I could lower it in the morning.

That night I was woken by thunder. From this high vantage point I had a good view of the lightening. But the semi-sitting-up position wasn't comfortable so I tried to lower the head. In the dark, I couldn't get the controls to work, so, to see what button was what, I switched the light on.

Beds I have known

Being high doesn't always improve visibility.

(Fortunately, it switches with a string pull so was still within reach.) But the light didn't come on. A few more tugs on the string. No light! I realized there must be a power-cut. So there I was, somewhere near the ceiling, dangerously high above the floor, out of earshot of help, out of reach of whistle. Trapped!

There was nothing for it, but to go back to sleep and hope the world would look less hopeless in the light of morning. It usually does. In fact, fortune smiled. At least I assume she must have, because the electricity came back on and I was able to lower the bed. By now, however, I was even less sure the bed was my friend. Somewhat later, when studying the control panel, I discovered my bed was model number 007. Now I was sure I couldn't trust it!

Lesson to be learnt: before making any ascent, always make sure you know the way down.

Much as I appreciated a harder mattress, difficulty rolling over meant I didn't do it often so my hip and shoulder would ache by morning. The nurse brought me a polythene air-mattress. This was delightfully soft - just like sleeping on bubble-wrap. `*Just like*'- indeed it looked and squeaked exactly like bubble-wrap! This made it quite noisy and *very* sweaty.

One night I was awakened by fog-horns. Fog-horns? I live five miles from the sea, even more till it's deep enough for any ship with brains. My cat was on the bed. Next-door-cat astride the window-sill. Clearly they didn't like each other. I added my voice to my cat's. I didn't speak cat-language (in fact, I can't howl at all), but next-door-cat understood and left - but not without a murderous "I'll be back" look. My cat was delighted, and to celebrate her victory, made a nest on the bed, pushing and pulling with her claws, and purring as cats do. In the morning, my bubble-wrap mattress was flat.

Lesson to be learnt: Fog-horns mean trouble. Cats mean trouble. Bubble-wrap means packaging. Fog-horns, cats and packaging have nothing to do with each other, so shouldn't be put together.

This wasn't the only bed I've had problems with. In one place I worked, my client put me up on a sofa-bed. Normally, to turn over, I must winch my body from one side to the other before rolling. This, however, was wide enough to let me roll without having to wake up completely. Being a fold-away design, it had a steel frame round its perimeter. This kept the edge high, but allowed the centre

Beds I have known

to sag. Advantage: it kept me in bed all night; no chance of falling out - this was good. Disadvantage: it also kept me in in the mornings - not so good! I would get to the edge, swing my legs out, lever myself up to sit to the edge - and roll back to the centre of the bed. This didn't hurt. Indeed it was fun - the first time. Much less fun by the fifth attempt. Eventually, however, I did manage to escape my (luxuriously soft) prison - and even developed a technique. Nonetheless, I never managed it at first try! Beyond being not-fun, however, there were other problems: I always start the day by sitting on the bed edge to pee into a bottle. This made rolling back even less fun. Holding a full pee bottle, it was definitely much less fun.

Lesson to be learnt: never get into anything you can't get out of.

Even harder was a friend's bed. This was low and soft. Very comfortable, but when I sat on the edge, I sunk into the mattress and found I was now too low to get up. My friends had, by now, left the house, so what started as something amusing was now a problem. Would I get to my medical appointment or just stay in bed all day? After innumerable failed attempts, I took a risk and rolled out, rolled across the floor (I can't crawl) to an armchair and managed to climb up it. It worked! But how many more times is fortune prepared to smile?

Lesson to be learnt: soft luxury is pleasant – but can be hard to break free from. Indeed, neither in bog, bed or life does it always help get you where you want to go.

Another problem bed was one I stayed in, in France. Arriving late at night, we found the bed only inches above the floor. A quick test proved I could never get out unaided. The house owner was out, but my friend found a rope. But what to fix it to? The only thing we could find was the door handle, but when I pulled, the latch clicked and the door swung open. Take up the rope slack and try again. This time, I managed to rise off the bed but thereafter could only swing around wildly. It being 4 a.m., we now gave up and I went to bed, accepting that I would have to wait for late-rising help the next (actually later in the same) morning. That day, we found bricks and raised the bed - though not quite enough!

The problems with Not-quite-high-enough-bed were not over, however. It had a mattress slightly wider than its frame. This made rolling over easier. But it also meant, when one morning I rolled over to look at the clock, that I suddenly found myself lying on it. Try as I might, I couldn't get back into bed - though I did manage to almost pull it off its bricks. Not knowing what the time was (How could I? I was lying on it) I didn't know whether it would be polite to call for help. Too early would be rude. Too late would mean waiting till the house-owner came home in the evening. Clearly, there was only a narrow help-window, but without a visible clock, I didn't know when this would be. True:

Beds I have known

I could feel the clock, but I couldn't see it. Fortunately, about an hour later, I heard someone in the kitchen and was able to make myself heard - and got rescued!

Lesson to be learnt: sometimes watching the clock doesn't help you rise in the world.

At one house I stayed in after a lecture, the bed was high. It was built over a cupboard - an excellent use of space, and definitely not too low to get up from. But I could see it would be a problem: could I get into it? Was there anywhere else I could sleep? Unfortunately, there wasn't.

Fortunately, however, I could - with some ingenuity - get into bed. Once in, the bed was quite comfortable. It was also good and solid - unlike a water-bed I once slept in. Although 'healthy' at that time, I had a cough. Coughing is not advisable in a water-bed; it makes waves. Result: by morning I felt sea-sick.

The real problem was one I had not anticipated: getting out. This was exacerbated by me. Walking on two sticks at that time, I knew I couldn't handle much luggage. I therefore took the minimum: toothbrush, coat, spare nappy, lecture slides and something to work on in the train. Hence - for lightness - no pajamas. The initial getting-out-of-bed was no problem, but the floor was slippery. The more I wriggled, the further my feet slipped and the less would they come back. Soon I was at forty-five degrees. What was more: I was blocking the door. What was even more: I had a train to catch. What was more again: I was naked, so too embarrassed to call for help. Fortunately, my elderly landlady did hear my ineffectual scrabbling, did manage to get in the door and did rescue me; and I did catch the train. Even more fortunately: she didn't tell me what she thought.

Lesson to be learnt: it may be nice to look down on the world, but isn't always so easy when you come down.

Another bed, in another friend's house, had a door problem. Beds don't usually have anything to do with doors, but this was a problem not with the bed itself, but with the front-door. It didn't close properly so in the middle of the night - when all good front-doors should be locked - opened silently. A neighbour noticed and phoned the police. The first I knew about this was a torch shone in my eyes. I'm not sure if it was meant to, but this woke me. The room was full of burly men in orange coats. Half-asleep, I couldn't work out what was happening. They asked me various questions. As I had just flown in late the previous night and, now only half-awake, didn't know where I was, I gave incoherent and unconvincing replies. Eventually I must have said something to upset them, because they left. Later, I realised that they were policemen. Even later, that they must have thought me a burglar. What a stupid idea! Even I know I'm not. But then some policemen can't even spell: they write 'ƎƆIꞀOԀ' on their cars. It took me, still quarter-asleep, even longer to realize that they were hunting *concealed* burglars. Apparently, resourceful burglars jump into

Beds I have known

bed whenever the police come. Really resourceful ones take a bundle of clothes with them to put beside the bed as evidence that they are asleep. Few, however, are resourceful enough to bring walking-sticks. Indeed, few people, and very few burglars, use them in bed.

Lesson to be learnt: when going to bed, always take everything you need with you. Especially if you expect company.

At a clinic I stayed in, I was put in a really fancy bed. Like mine at home, it went up, down, folded and sandwiched. Unlike mine (after de-construction), it had a monkey pole. This, however, didn't fit the bed, so had to be tied on with bandages. (Nurses are resourceful.) So far, so good. Only an alarming sway and resounding clang whenever I pulled on it. If I raised the bed, however, the monkey pole would stay put, while my nose would rise into the handle directly above it. Perhaps one reason monkeys have flat noses?

On the next visit, I got a matching bed-and-pole set. This bed also had 'safety' sides. Being fenced in, I couldn't get out without assistance, so was given a nurse-call switch on a cable. But where could this go and be within reach? Hung from the monkey-pole handle of course! Where could the lift/tilt/sandwich bed-controller go? Likewise, hung from the monkey-pole handle. And the pull-cord for the light? This too. This made three strings and cables over my head. If I needed to roll over during the night, all I needed do was reach up, carefully feed my hand between them, pull on the handle to lift myself, and roll. One of these strings, however, was connected to the light. This meant that every pull on the monkey-pole, for whatever purpose, would always switch it on. The monkey-pole may have eased rolling over, but was, therefore, no help to getting quickly back to sleep. Worse than this: if the surprise caused me to jerk upright, my head would pass through the three string and cable entanglement. This would not be my chosen way of hanging from a monkey-pole.

Lesson to be learnt: be careful when choosing bed-partners. There can be unintended consequences. And even the easiest ones often come with strings.

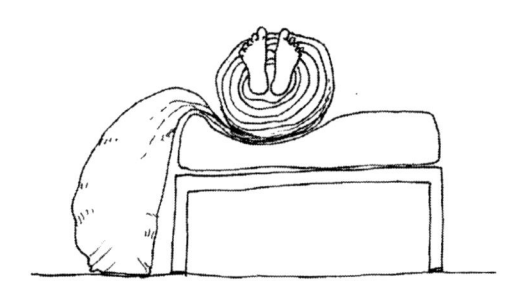

Hospital mattresses are hygienic – namely plastic.
Fortunately, incontinence is impossible: I sweat all liquids out.
Unfortunate result: the sheets – but not duvet contents – stick to me when I roll over.

8. Chairs I Trust; Chairs I Don't Trust

Sitting is easy. Not so sitting down. Standing up even less so. With soft sofas, if I make a mistake while sitting down, I know I can just fall the last bit. But how can I get up? The more I press with one arm the more this just sinks in - leaving me stuck. Without company, soft sofas are no fun.
Lesson to be learnt: soft sofas are best with a friend.

My own sofa is higher and harder. But unless I can get to the wall end and pull myself up on the radiator, I can't get up. Rolling along the sofa is hazardous. As I'm not perfectly cylindrical, I drift outwards when rolling, so risk rolling off. For safety, therefore, I had a rope fixed to the beams to pull on. To give better grip this rope was knotted with loops. In these I could also hang my crutches, so that they would be within reach, not fallen on the floor, when I did finally manage to get up. This seemed a good idea, but unfortunately the end result looked too much like a hangman's noose. Hanging from a noose - whether deliberate or by accident - would not be a good idea. It takes all the pleasure out of watching television.

Lesson to be learnt: body shape matters - especially when rolling along sofas.

Now I have an electric armchair. It isn't actually mine. The Motor Neurone Society leant it to me, so I must return it when I die. (I still haven't quite worked out how I can do this.) This chair reclines luxuriously, even putting feet up to table level for maximum sprawl-comfort. Hence it's usually occupied by a teenager. It also rises and tilts so as to tip me onto my feet – or onto the floor if my legs don't cooperate. The controls are simple: two buttons, one up, one down. Even I could learn to operate this in less than a day. But where to put the controller? I like to hang it on the right side, where I can reach it. But others usually leave it in the chair. This means I sit on it and can't find it. Not only that, but my bottom operates it. Hence the chair, dutifully obeying bottom-commands, moves inexorably to the eject position or, if I'm luckier, the recline position. Here, however, with my full body weight on the controller there is no chance I can reach it.

Lesson to be learnt: watch TV with a friend.

I also have an office chair on wheels. This was given to me by the government. (Governments also play the two policeman trick. This was the 'nice policeman' bit of the government.) Wheels means it moves easily around the room. It does this whether I want it to or not. Sneezing, for instance, propels me backwards. Sitting down transfers a vertical load into a horizontal force, so shoots the chair back across the room. I must then jiggle chair and myself until I can reach furniture on which to haul myself back to where I want to be.

A further problem is that I don't actually own the chair. On paper, it is the government's. In reality, it is the cat's. Cats add hazard here. My cat knows it is *her* chair. (Actually I don't own her, she owns me - and isn't even sure if I deserve to be owned.) I only *think* it is mine. But she *knows* it is hers. To sit, I carefully lower myself down, but she won't get up from it. What she doesn't know, but I do, is that there is a point of no return beyond which I can't halt my seating process. She still doesn't move. So I have to sit on the front edge, leaving the warm rear to her. If, as is often the case, the tilt-lock is loose, this means I tip forward and the chair rockets back, eventually crashing into something. Fortunately, this always gets rid of the cat. Unfortunately, it sometimes also gets rid of me.

Getting up can be a major challenge. I raise myself on the arms, lean forward, then start to straighten my legs. Half-straight legs mean half-horizontal force. At this point, therefore, the chair moves backwards, so necessitating a quick decision: Can I complete standing? If not I'll sit back down in the space where the chair was - but now isn't. I'm rarely brave enough to risk this, so I just hold on and wait to see where the now accelerating chair takes me.

Naturally I have developed a technique for getting out of Office Chair - otherwise, I would still be in it. I hold the underside of my desk and pull myself up. When my fingers slip, however, if unlucky, I find myself on the floor, the chair waiting patiently behind me. If lucky, I'm safely mounted on the chair, but in the middle of the room, no finger holds in reach....

Lesson to be learnt: getting up off one's bottom is important. If you can't do it right, expect to go downhill fast.

Additional lesson to be learnt: as in life, always have something solid behind you. This (or she, or he) should not be fragile.

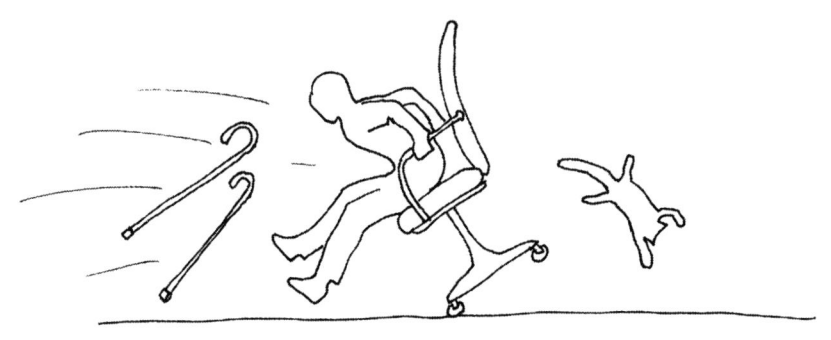

High-speed cat removal.

I now have Electric Office Chair. This is big, black and looks disquietingly like an all-plastic dentist's couch, 1980's style. Actually, when it arrived, it was in the full-recline and table-height-raised position, so looked *exactly* like one. As well as its dental-couch function, it can do everything you might need - or not need - in an office: rise to close to ceiling height, pivot, turn, recline and eject.

Chairs I Trust; Chairs I Don't Trust

(This last is useful for dealing with cats.) At least, I thought it would do all this - if it worked. It arrived with two instruction books. One - in English, Norwegian, Swedish and Finnish - about how to use the chair. One - about technical information - in German, French, Dutch and Italian. In the European age, this naturally presumes a bi-lingual office - or anyway a bi-lingual cripple. The handbook promises a "thrilling outdoor ride". Until I read this, I had wondered what cripples do in offices that requires headlights, horn and flashing hazard lights.

One instruction told me to disconnect the batteries if the chair wouldn't be used for a period. It obviously hadn't been, because they were already disconnected. Nowhere, however, did it describe how to *re*-connect them. It did advise me to get a service engineer from head office - in Sweden. As the government had arranged it, I contacted them instead. As it had only taken five months to arrive from first being ordered, I shouldn't have been surprised that nothing happened for another two. My son was much more helpful. Being a teenager, he naturally knew all about such things, so tried three different ways of reconnection - each accompanied by dramatic blue flashes and loud bangs. Eventually, I persuaded him that one disabled person in the house was enough; also that the chair - if it ever worked - would be more useful in one piece than in thousands, embedded in the ceiling, walls, him and me. Clearly the machine was powerful, but until we knew *what* to do with it, just ate up space. Not everyone wants a dentist's couch in their home. Nor, even though I normally appreciate all free gifts, did I.

Lesson to be learnt: knowledge without power doesn't go anywhere.

Eventually we found someone to connect the various bits and make the chair live - or anyway, make it work. It now rises, lowers, tips and folds; leg-rests rise and fall - all accompanied by bestial groans and snarls from the malevolent force hidden within. Unfortunately, its road-manners leave much to be desired. It doesn't like to stop. More precisely, it *will* stop, but not when I tell it to. Its motor responds to all commands after about one second's delay. Momentum then carries it a bit further again. I don't mind stopping late – this shows it's not work-shy - but when I'm trying to get close, but not *too* close, to my desk, my knees mind.

This is a serious, painful and cripple-the-cripple disadvantage. But the chair has some advantages too. It gives a unique distinction to any office. And it certainly looks impressive - in a Star Wars, Evil Empire-ish sort of way. Indeed, its looks were too much for one of my carers. She couldn't resist pushing at the buttons. When it squeaked and the lights flashed on, she jumped back in horror, pulling at the little control lever to stop it. As this lever is, in fact, an accelerator, far from stopping the chair, it started it. As she backed off, but didn't let go, so she pulled the lever towards herself. Result: however much she dodged,

Chairs I Trust; Chairs I Don't Trust

the chair pursued her round the room with uncanny accuracy. It isn't funny - in fact it's a bit frightening - to be chased by a chair. Especially one dressed up like Darth Vader.

With its sinister all-black PVC outfit and sadistic habits, I'm not convinced Electric Office Chair is a friend. As I don't trust it, it's currently unemployed. Not surprisingly, this makes it resentful. At the moment, it just sits in the corner of the office, glowering.

Lesson to be learnt: power without knowledge is a dangerous beast.

9. Domestic Staff

Being ill means giving some things up. I used to enjoy cooking, cooked all the meals and baked most of the bread. As my mobility, stability and dexterity deteriorated, I had to give up cooking and my (now ex-) wife had to do it. This was too much! Being cook turned her from a professional woman to a 'housewife' - the worst insult possible. She left, taking our two-year-old with her. The less said about this the better. The one good thing is she is now ex. And the lesson to be learnt? Don't get ill - it's unhealthy.

But there remained practical problems - not least: the need for food. Food is useful - so useful, it's nice to have some every day, not just a huge mound once a week.

My daughter came to help, but she herself was unwell, so I needed to hire a cook. I needed help with other things too, like bed-making, laundry, cleaning, reaching things... an endless list. Overnight I became an employer - by (extreme left) definition: a capitalist exploiter of the underpaid. Just as well I never joined the Trotskyist Revolutionary Party of the People's Proletariat in my youth. Actually, I couldn't. I could never understand what dyslexic materialism meant (or was it: dielectric materialism? or dyspeptic materialism?). Politics were never my strong point: another political term I had trouble with was 'polemic'. I know *what* it means: polly (from parrot) and emic (from emetic), but not what this has to do with politics. Or, at least, I *hope* I don't know.

I decided to employ cook and carer separately, so they could fill in for each other if one went on holiday. This made me a major employer. Fortunately, of the many pairs, always there was one responsible enough to give two months notice before going away. Unfortunately, the other - less responsible - one would invariably go away at the same time, giving only one day's notice. So much for contingency planning!

Too (even two) many people also brings coordination problems. I now have one person who cooks - and fills the compost bucket; one who makes my bed - and puts the hot-water-bottle and cover beside the compost bucket; one who fills the bottle and puts it in my bed, thoughtfully setting my pajamas to warm on it. And none who empties the compost. Result: happy ants in kitchen. Further result: ants, when taking tea-break, snooze inside hot-water-bottle cover. Even further result: ants in bed - and in pajamas. As an animal lover, I shouldn't mind. But one result of being ill - and having carers put ants in my bed - is that I look at things differently now.

Lesson to be learnt: too many cooks (and carers) cause ants in pants.

Even single cooks, however, aren't problem-free. Quite naturally, every cook wants to make the kitchen 'her own'. This means each cook in turn re-arranges things - not *everything*, only about three-quarters of everything. Moreover, each cook knows better than her predecessor exactly where I *ought* to want things - or perhaps they are just competing in ingenuity. Even the best cooks, and even the ones I get on with really well, only stay about a year - they've too many talents to just spend their time cooking. Unfortunately the worst cooks also stay about a year. This isn't good for the stomach. The net result, however, is that once three-quarters of everything has been re-arranged several times (a different three-quarter selection each time), when a new cook asks me where something is, I only know where it *was*. I'm not sure how much this helps.

Carers like re-arranging too. After all, *they* know where things are, even if they leave a few weeks later. Between cooks and carers, this means I own lots of things that can't be found, so need to be re-bought. And re-bought again… and again… This makes me a major property owner. Also, it must be good for the national economy, but isn't good for mine. Nonetheless, all the manufacturing this economic growth entails is clearly not sustainable.

Lesson to be learnt. Dying is not sustainable; you can't keep on doing it for ever.

Cooks and carers have been varied. Some were excellent, some cheated, stole and lied. Some couldn't cook and some didn't care. Some shouldn't have ever been allowed to even try to cook. I began to understand the common gripe: "You just can't get good staff these days!"

Interviewing prospective cooks, I learnt that people know a lot about food. Indeed the weirder their diet, the more definitively do they know what is good for me. Vegans, raw-foodists, sprouters, high-protein carnivores, macro-biots, nutters, seedy-weedies and juicy-woosies all know what is good and that everything else is poison. But these are just ordinary un-common diets. Weird dietists know this ten times better. Unfortunately I never knew this - and after some of that food, don't want to ever know it.

One cook, in particular, was vegan. Honest, responsible, resourceful, inventive, but vegan. Being vegetarian for half my life, I know vegan food can be delicious, but for this cook, it wasn't only no meat, no fish, no eggs, no milk, but also no salt, no sugar, no wheat, no yeast and, as I learnt, no herbs, no flavour, no experience of cooking and no sense of humour. With so many NOs, I began to wonder whether he liked, or hated, food.

Domestic Staff

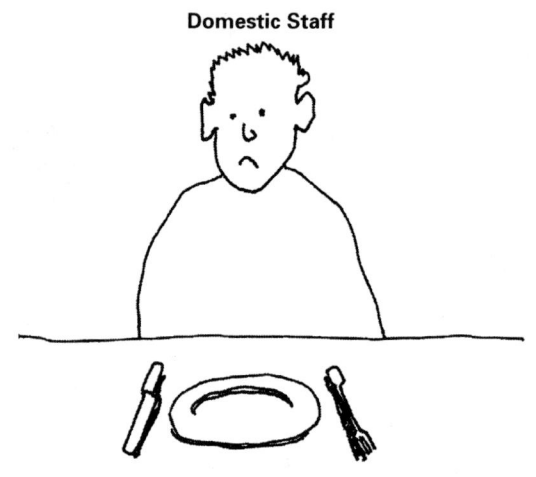

From food experts, it's best not to ask for a second opinion.
There ends up being nothing you can eat.

It's well known that too much salt is bad for you, but absolutely *no* salt upsets the body's saline balance causing, in my case, muscle cramps at night. (Anyone who thinks foot cramps are painful, should try calf cramps. If you think these are bad, try thigh cramps!) Also, when food is boiled without *any* salt at all, osmosis ensures that all flavour - and with it most nutrition - passes from the food to the water. If you hate food, this may be alright, but not otherwise. However expensive the ingredients, all food tastes of nothing. Actually, not *all* food tasted of nothing because the cook liked to experiment. Some experiments were unique. No-one else had ever thought of them - nor (hopefully) ever will. In the interests of public health, some should be included in a list of recipes to avoid. These include:

Mashed potato without butter, milk or salt, only water and peanut-butter.

Bread-and-butter pudding without butter, milk or sugar - ingredients: bread, water, five raisins.

Soup made from nut-loaf leftovers; the nut-loaf in turn based on macaroni-cheese leftovers (being cheese-free, this was actually: macaroni, soy-milk and cornflower). To ensure it wasn't too thin (or nutty or not-cheesy), it was further thickened with water-mashed potato (made to the unique recipe I was now - unfortunately - beginning to get used to).

Millet and mayonnaise blended to a pulp, served as cold salad.

Swede and mushroom stew (rubbery texture of mushrooms, but taste: only swede).

Garlic and carrot juice (equal parts)

Curried beetroot juice. This so burned my throat, that I couldn't speak to complain!

As a vegan he didn't know that raw eggs go bad - how could he?

Domestic Staff

This meant mayonnaise ('keep refrigerated after opening') left on the table for me day and night for three hot months of summer. I never finished the jar. It wasn't very appealing on the first day and appealed less on each subsequent day. Being wheat-free, he didn't know bread is only nice fresh, so, like the mayonnaise, it stayed on the table day after day. Just like the mayonnaise, the less I ate, the more patiently it waited. When I explained to him that bread gets stale, he thanked me and thereafter carefully wrapped the bread in polythene. Result: after four days, it wasn't bread but fur.

There was also 'safer' vegan food like vegan chicken breasts - or were they fish fillets? Anyway, that's what they looked like. On the plate there was no label to say what they were (chicken, fish, vegan chicken [the kind that only eats grain], or mystery ingredient). Nor, being filleted, was it possible to tell from the bones. Certainly I couldn't from the flavour - there was none. Retrospectively, I now assume they were chicken-fish textured soya fillets.

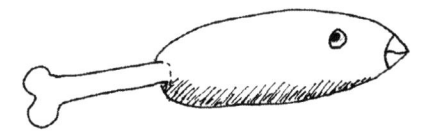

Vegan chicken-fish cutlet.

He also cooked more conventional food, like quiche. This was healthy, its pastry base in particular: wholemeal flour with minimal, if any, margarine. As the whole thing was made and cooked within the hour he allotted for supper preparation, the eggy top was almost raw, so indigestible. The base, however, being one inch thick, was sufficiently filling even when uncooked. One disarmingly small diameter quiche was more than enough for four people and the dog.

Gradually I succeeded in educating him in the things I can't eat, but not without feeling nauseous after almost every meal. Result: more and more supermarket instant meals. These used to make me feel sick - and still I do. I never dreamt I would so appreciate them! Likewise, when I had physiotherapy, occupational therapy and speech therapy at the hospital, between the hours of vacant waiting came hospital lunch: sausages, mashed potato, vegetable sludge and gravy - what bliss!

Fortunately, he left for a better job: cooking for an invalid with digestive problems. Unfortunately, I understand that she is now dead.

Lesson to be learnt: ask prospective cooks if they like or hate food. Also ask if they've ever cooked before.

Further lesson to be learnt: life is good, but food isn't always.

Since then I've interviewed other cooks (and would-be cooks and obviously would-not-be-cooks). I've now learnt that no meat, no fish, no eggs, no milk, no

Domestic Staff

wheat, no oven experience (and there are surprisingly many such who want to cook for me - and even want to be paid for it) means: no job.

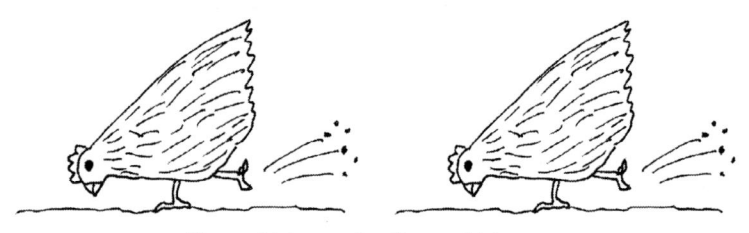

Vegan chicken and ordinary chicken.
The difference: one worm.

Carers, likewise, have varied from the excellent to the young, beautiful (and dishonest). This one spent most of her time avoiding the advances of my apprentice, and the rest either making tea or disappearing. I would overhear conversations like: Apprentice: "Today is my birthday. I would like to do something special tonight. I would like to spend it with you." Carer (to me): "Would you like a cup of tea?" Sound of electric kettle. But no tea, no carer - not till the next morning. And possibly - or not(?) - no special night.

This carer was very willing to help with extra-mural things like selling semi-antiques - although they never actually got sold. Or did they? She also did do *some* work, and at this she seemed amazingly efficient and quick. After she disappeared, however, (not dead or abducted by aliens, but subsequently found working in a pub - and owing me semi-antique money) I discovered 'filing' meant putting things out of sight. *Where* and whether they could ever be found again was apparently not important. How can I protect myself from future theft? I'm not sure what *I* can do, but it would certainly help if the government made crime illegal.

Lesson to be learnt: learn the Buddhist art of non-attachment *before* things (and employees with them) go missing. Not *after.*

Further lesson to be learnt: chose truth before beauty (in an employee; in a politician, expect neither. So never employ a politician as a cook or carer.)

Another carer did everything at high speed. Whatever, or however unpleasant, the job, she worked with such goodwill and enthusiasm that she did four times as much as work in the time it would take anyone else. But each job was only three-quarters finished. This still meant she did three times as much, so I could hardly complain. Unfortunately, however, it is only completion that makes a job worth starting.

Lesson to be learnt: a job three-quarter done wasn't really worth doing at all. Is this a lesson for life? Is a life three-quarter lived worth living? Is living without dying really worth the hassle?

10. Bio-hazards: Living with Teenagers and Other Animals

Cats

Cats may look sweet, but they're dangerous. Dangerous to mice. Dangerous to cripples like me. Especially dangerous are friendly cats. The hungrier they are, the friendlier – and more deadly. Friendly cats like to rub on legs. They rub sideways and then push up with their heads. As cats like to be noticed, it doesn't take them long to work out that lifting crutches off the floor is more effective than trying to lift legs. I certainly notice when the crutch is lifted - without friction contact with the floor, it slips. Some cats are smart enough to realize that rubbing their backs on crutches *always* gets results. Hence when these are leant against a table, they get the same rub-a-crutch treatment. Result: crutch on floor, cat affronted by near-miss, and me marooned. This may not get cat breakfast, but it does learn some non-dictionary words. There remains, of course, the problem of how to pick up crutch. If I can hold onto something, I can probably get it. If not, I'm both marooned *and* sunk - a bad combination. (For this reason I'm working on a magnetic-crutch invention. Unfortunately, there are problems. Apart from the weight of steel - which affects balance - crutches that spring together aren't easy to walk with.)

Between rubbing crutches, their behaviour is more normal, just walking between my legs, trying successfully to get noticed by each foot in turn. (This is one of the few habits cats share with dogs. When, in healthier times, I walked in a field with a bull in, I found bulls don't like dogs. In fact, they want to chase them. Dogs don't like being chased by bulls. So, for security, dog likes to hide between my legs. This is not the most popular thing a dog can do.)

Lesson to be learnt: living creatures aren't welcome between the legs.

Unfriendly cats can also cause problems. One house I stayed in had an unfriendly-cat kind of cat problem. Naturally, the owners thought the cat friendly and lovable. I was less sure. The bedroom and toilet were upstairs. Not an uncommon arrangement, but for me it meant several high-risk adventures a day. With great care, I could grip the stair balusters and sidle slowly up- or down- stairs. But resident-tom-cat liked to sleep in the sun on the landing. Sleeping all day is boring, so for entertainment, he liked to roll over and leisurely sink his claws into my hand grasping the balustrade. This didn't really hurt, but nor did it make life easy. Normally, when play-hooked by cats, you just push towards cat to disengage claws, then smartly remove hand and, from position of safety, educate cat in use of extended vocabulary. (Cats learn a lot of English this way - or anyway, a few short words a lot of times.) That's the normal way to extricate oneself from naughty cats. But no longer being so stable, I didn't dare let go of handrail, so couldn't get out of range. This restricted my vocabulary. As I was often alone in the house, I became rather nervous of going upstairs.

This in turn affected how much I dared drink. In such ways, cats have an effect on health.

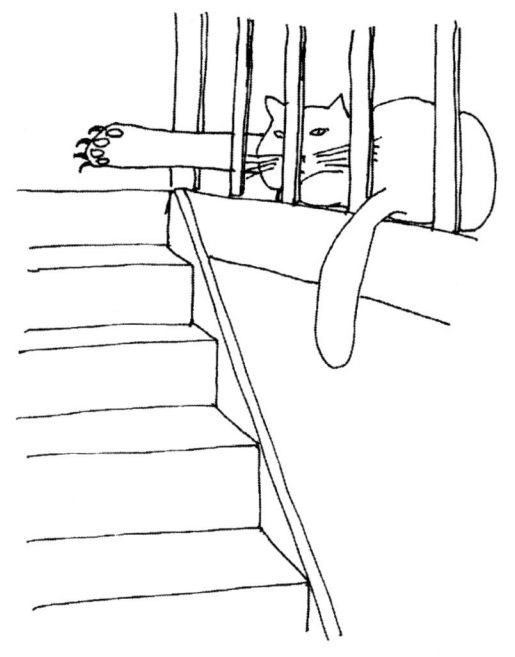

Cat-guard home protection.

Dogs

Apart from French kissing hazards, friendly dogs like to show you how important they are. To do this, they have to push past - usually on steps, steep slippery paths or other such well-chosen places. Walking also requires extra care in doggyland. Often the exact spot I need to place my crutch or drag my foot to, has been claimed as a depository of that (copious) less pleasant side of dogs (Dogs' Gift to Mankind).

My neighbour's dog is crossed with a doormat – from which he inherited his brains – if any. Like doormats, he is always where I want to step next. He is however, bright enough to recognize that he's in the wrong place, so he turns - usually towards me - quite unaware, or unconcerned, that he's pushing me over. What does that matter to a doormat!

Little Yappers are less popular. Sudden yaps can make me jump. Dogs that like sticks, likewise have limited popularity. Some will grab any stick, including walking sticks. Unfortunately, stick-popularity isn't limited to wood. It also means attraction to teeth-splintering crutches, so on the beach I attract many new four-footed friends and not-so-friends. Some are so friendly that they want to lick my mouth - these are usually bigger, heavier and sometimes even stupider than me. Others take offence - usually at the crutches, occasionally at me.

Bio-hazards: Living with Teenagers and Other Animals

For safety therefore, I adopt the three-point brace position and wait till their interest, affection or hostility has passed. Unfortunately however, some dogs regard every motionless metal pole as a territory marker, which doggy convention obliges them to mark.

Lesson to be learnt: friendliness without brains is a mixed blessing; unfriendliness with brains, a mixed curse.

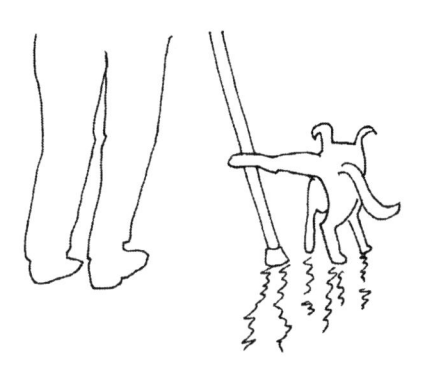

Dogs may be friendly, but crutches slip on wet ground.

Teenagers

Living with teenagers presents special problems. I'm glad they are able to cook, because this supplements all the easy food that disappears from the larder faster than it can be stacked on shelves. I know they can cook, because I constantly hear the microwave and there is a permanent greasy bit of floor near the stove with a few escaped oven-ready chips sleeping in it. (I know they sleep, because they never get up.) This grease-patch is lethal for crutches - and if I'm not careful, lethal for me.

I have learnt never to hurry for the phone when it rings. Firstly, because the grease-patch needs five-minute negotiation, secondarily because I'm unlikely to reach the phone in time and thirdly, because it's never there, but under something in a teenager's bedroom. Fortunately none of my children are to blame for wandering telephone, dead chips or grease - nor indeed anything else. They've "never seen", nor touched, anything. This is true. I know their amazing skill at doing things while half-asleep. If I do try to blame someone, or - even worse - ask them to do something, this definitely "isn't fair." As they've never seen the missing phone, I feel quite OK about pressing the handset-locator button - which causes the phone to shriek its whereabouts - even at inconsiderately early hours, like noon. It may be deathly quiet up there in teenager-land, but they're not dead. Every so often they need me to be a walking (in my case, hobbling) cash-machine or instant taxi. In the afternoons, however, teenagers become audible - indeed they're audible over a two-mile radius. (Actually, even a single teenager is usually triply audible: radio, CD player and amplified guitar,

Bio-hazards: Living with Teenagers and Other Animals

each playing different music.) This continues until early morning. (They are, after all a nocturnal species.)

Lesson to be learnt: need diminishes with age. The younger you are, the more you *need* things – and need them *immediately*. The older - or more disabled - you are, the less you get them - if at all! Hence, as you can live without them, you obviously didn't need them.

From advertisements, I should have already learnt that I shouldn't need things. After all, if I could survive for years without 'indispensable' things, I ought to be able to dispense with 'ordinary' ones. I should also have learnt that the longer you live, the longer you have done without things, so the longer you can wait. I *should* have learnt this, but I'm still asking God to give me patience – NOW!

Of course, there are also things teenagers (or if not them, possibly it was the cat) borrow, with or without my knowledge. Some, they even put back. But teenagers have long arms and can reach things. I can't. I must have everything I need within reach. Four more inches away, and I can probably reach it. Eight, and I will probably fall out of my chair in the attempt. Twelve, and I am certain it isn't worth trying. This makes me unreasonably fussy about where things are - so confirming the younger generation view that older people are up-tight.

Lesson to be learnt: seized muscles easily make you up-tight.

One surprising thing about teenagers is how many suddenly become interested in gardening. This is good, because I can no longer get to the garden to grow vegetables. Actually, they don't grow vegetables but flowers. One particular spiky-leafed one seems to be in fashion. I've never seen this in flower, however. Just when the plants get fully tall, the slugs always wipe out the whole crop.

Lesson to be learnt: Gardening has a calming influence.

Slugs

Slugs move slower than me - but this doesn't stop them ambushing me. They have been known to wait all night in the middle of the floor for me to tread on them. This is squidgy. As it doesn't feel very nice in bare feet, I recommend wearing boots in slug country. It's much more serious when they position themselves for my crutches. This is slippery - and could be fatal. Crutch-slip is a major hazard in disabled life. What have I ever done to slugs, that they would want to kill me?

Lesson to be learnt: never trust a slug.

Midges

Midges are faster than me. This isn't fair. This means that whereas some people go for a walk to feed ducks, I go for a walk to feed midges. There's no way I can out-run, out-fly, out-walk or even out-hobble them. I can't wave a tail like a horse, or wave a crutch like a semi-cripple. Nor can I wipe them off my face mid-bite or even scratch post-bite. If I try any of this I would fall. And that is worse than being bitten because, supine, I can't run away, so get bitten more. In fact I would get bitten and bitten until they - and all their friends - were bored. Unfortunately it's very hard to bore a midge. Unfortunately again, they know all this and take advantage. This is very unfair advantage. As every midge I've ever met does this, I can only conclude that midges aren't fair. Maybe life isn't fair.

Lesson to be learnt: never expect compassion from a midge.

11. Surviving Architecture: non-accessible accessibility

Architecture: Ancient and Modern

Modern architecture may be 'disabled accessible', but it's often gracefully smooth. Indeed, the more modern, the smoother. It seems that, to prove their modernity, many architects enter an unofficial smoothness competition. This may look nice, but, personally, I never feel safe with smoothies – especially underfoot.

Smooth floors mean taking my life in my hands (in this case: not hands, but feet). Walking with sticks, now crutches, I need these to stay on the bit of floor I put them on. Smooth floors are slippery - especially when they, or the stick ferrule - are wet. I therefore always plant my stick on the joint *between* tiles, or against protruding nail-heads, floor-wall junction or some such place. Some floors are too smooth to have joints. For me, these are lake-like barriers – as calm and safe-looking, but as dangerous to swim across with crutches.

Fortunately few older buildings are so suave. Unfortunately, they too aren't immune to the shiny-gloss treatment, turning tolerable surfaces into frighteningly slippery ones. Wood floors can be so mirror-varnished that they look and feel like plastic. (Actually, with enough polyurethane, they now *are*!) True: this helps me cover the floor fast. But I don't always *want* to cover the floor.

Generally, smoothifying floors is expensive for low-budget home-owners. They prefer carpets. Unfortunately, small carpets are cheaper than large ones. Mini-carpets are prone to the Magic Carpet Trick. Magic carpets (even mini-magic-carpets) don't just fly – they also transport you to another world. Unfortunately again, I'm not quite ready to pass on to this.

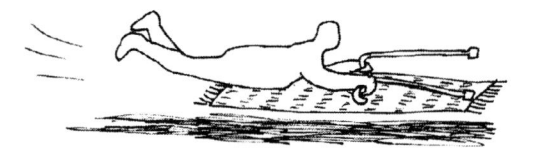

The flying carpet trick.

Walls aren't much better. In fact, I begin to wonder how many architects ever think about finger-holds. True: some not-quite-so-modern buildings have exposed brickwork with neatly raked joints. These give about quarter of an inch purchase, just enough for a little finger. Such scanty holds are only effective when reaching high or far to the side. Neither are good positions for balance – and, worse, I don't usually have a safety rope. Even worse, I don't make a very convincing spider-man.

In one hotel café, my helper went to deal with luggage, leaving me to finish breakfast and get up. But the seat was low, the table tipped when I pushed on it

Surviving Architecture: non-accessible accessibility

and the brickwork joints were just too shallow. Yes, I could finish breakfast - but how could I get up? Had she not come back to help, I would have had to stay to lunch.

Lesson to be learnt: immobility isn't good for the waistline.

Older buildings were never designed with disability in mind, so are usually richly supplied with steps and suchlike hazards. Fortunately, they're often also rich in the scars and abuses of history. At hazard-points, I'm always on the lookout for things to hold onto. Things like picture-rails, dados, damaged plaster, knot-holes, or even not-very-secure pipes and electrical cables clipped to walls. Fortunately, there are usually lots.

Unfortunately, some knot-holes won't let go of fingers. This can be very embarrassing – both for trapped spider-men and spiders trapped at home. Also, pipes and cables can be very sensitive. Injured pipes tend to get their own back. They can soak, scald, or - at the very least - becalm me in the centre of an ocean of slippery floor. Boiled spider-man risk. Nor is it so appealing to hold live-ended electric cables. If you let go, who knows whom the live end will touch. If you deliberately short it, to blow the fuse, you risk being blinded by the flash. Moreover, after blinding, you'll be trapped in total darkness, so won't be able to see anything. Ruptured gas-pipes have even greater dramatic potential. I have, however, never wanted to actually *be* part of a firework. This is fried spider-man risk.

Lesson to be learnt: sometimes you need some rough with the smooth.

The search for finger-holds often leads to the less solid parts of buildings. Where I'm confident the door won't close, I can put two fingers in the crack between door and frame, and cross them - as in rock-climbing - to jam them in. I'm also hoping the crossed fingers will bring me luck - specifically that the door won't shut and amputate them.

Important lesson: if planning to become disabled, learn rock-climbing.

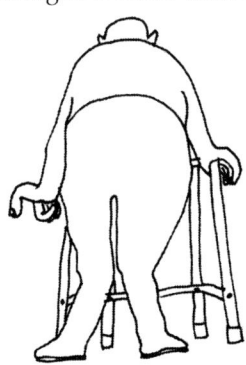

Being unable to rotate my left arm, I use my little finger to hold onto supports.
Advantage: super-strong little finger (good for rock-climbing).
Disadvantage: I look a little odd (not good for my modelling career).

Surviving Architecture: non-accessible accessibility

Over recent years there has been a general tendency for things to *look* good (and smooth), but not necessarily *be* solid. This is no help when rock-climb traversing around rooms. Smooth-lipped basins, flimsy towel rails, plastic hooks and handles, and lightweight furniture are the bane of the furniture-crawling disabled. True: there may be spiders *under* them, but this is no help for disabled-spider-man trainees.

Fortunately, most new buildings are bound by disability legislation. Unfortunately, most have been designed by people with disabled – or at least, abled-thinking - brains. If only they had experienced life from the disabled side! 'Disabled-accessible' buildings have handrails fitted in useful places like toilets. Handrails are very important for building permits. In the right place, they're also important for getting off the toilet. Often, however, they've been positioned by people who have never needed to use one (handrail, not toilet). When I sit on a toilet with the handrail behind my feet, I naturally appreciate the consideration, but even more naturally, I'm worried about how I'll ever pull myself past my centre of gravity. As I'm not the sort of person who enjoys being stuck for days in toilets, I always examine the escape routes, hand-holds and disability aids first. This is particularly necessary in 'disabled bathrooms' as some have (the only) handrail behind my head. These are useless: How could anyone with hands growing out of the back of their head even use a bathroom?

Lesson to be learnt: constipation aids include mis-located handrails.

Further lesson to be learnt: if in doubt, bring a good book.

Old furniture is reassuringly heavy; often so heavy it won't move however much you lean on it. As this means that *nobody* can move it, resourceful people fix on wheels. It now becomes at once solid *and* highly mobile – a bit like a tank with the brakes off. As one such sofa killed my grandmother, I'm cautious of such military vehicles. Nor am I that keen on fashionable furniture. Some is graceful but flimsy. Some just flimsy. This means it can't be relied upon if I want to steady myself on it, but can be relied on to expensively break if I fall on it.

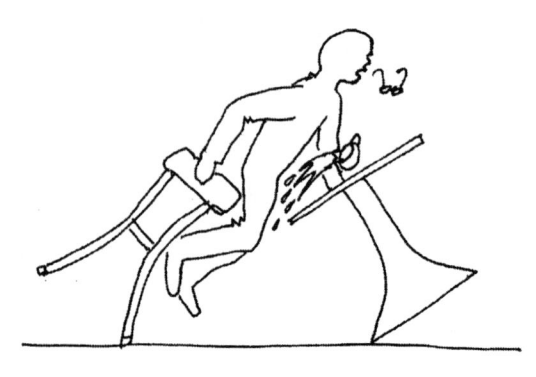

Coffee sandwich.

Surviving Architecture: non-accessible accessibility

In one café, the only free seating was on bar stools. Bar-stools require you to hop backwards up onto them. If you *climb* up them, using the foot-rest as a step, they capsize - as I discovered. I may be slow, but fortunately I was quick enough to grab onto the table to save myself from falling. Unfortunately the table was also fashionable. It too capsized, but the opposite way. This meant bar-stool and table closed like a trap around me. By this clever design stratagem my fall was slowed, so saving me from serious injury and the café from litigation to recover the cost of my lost coffee. I didn't exactly lose the coffee. In fact, it found me. Once I was safely on the floor, the contents of four cups rained on my stomach, followed by the cups themselves, then the saucers, then four cakes and lastly - as a considerate gesture - by four paper napkins.

Lesson to be learnt: coffee is best taken internally, not applied externally.

Ramps and Escalators

Lots of places provide ramps, escalators or lifts for the disabled. Escalators aren't easy. Should I hold onto the moving handrail and get pulled onto my nose? Or place one foot on the first step and have one leg pulled from under me before being tipped backwards? When only walking with one stick, I tried an 'easy' flat travelator. Never again! Laborious as they are, I prefer long walks, or even stairs.

Lesson to be learnt: even if you put your best foot forward, you may end up going into things head first.

Fortunately, some buildings don't depend on technological booby-traps like escalators or lifts. They just have ramps. As these are invariably afterthoughts, they are prone to suffer from afterthought syndrome. One particularly prestigious museum had a broad, gently graded ramp. But where was it? To find it, you had to climb the steep un-handrailed formal front-steps, then queue for twenty minutes to ask at the information counter. And, of course, go down the steps – counter-flow to people coming up - which, like all mountaineering descents, is more dangerous than the ascent.

Lesson to be learnt: plan all mountaineering routes carefully before starting.

Stair-Lifts

To meet disabled-accessibility obligations, many public buildings have retrofitted wheelchair stair-lifts. Not requiring structural changes to buildings, they're cheaper than proper lifts, hence popular with building owners. They're not, however, always so popular with me.

The British Medical Association offices have corridors with many short flights of steps, each with a stair-lift. With these, you stand on a platform, exactly the size of a wheelchair - no larger. You then fold down a handrail and press the start button. A savage jolt dispenses with anyone not disabled enough to need

Surviving Architecture: non-accessible accessibility

to hang on tight, then the platform shudders with agonizing slowness up its four-step climb. In twenty paces (sixty for me) comes another flight of steps and stair-lift. But which is the greater risk: stairs or stair-lift?

Not all stair-lifts are so rickety. One plush modern one in a plush modern sports centre ran silently and smoothly. But it was slow. So slow, I could easily cross to the handrail side of the stairs and climb them before it had even come down for me to get on. Clearly, the athletes who used this weren't sprinters. Nor was it for anyone needing a toilet in a hurry.

Lesson to be learnt: Avoid the most hazardous route, but when nature calls don't take the slowest either.

In one pre-disabled buildings the toilets were in the basement. Basements, however, aren't easy to get to in wheelchairs, or even on crutches. But chair-lift to the rescue! This one was a motorized chair hung off a sort of wall-mounted track alongside the stairs. All you had to do was sit in it and press a button. But to sit in it, you needed to take three steps down the stairs, turn - without a handrail to hold, because the chair is in the way - stand on one leg (the other being on the wrong step) and just sit in the chair. My friend tried it out. So far, so good; she managed to sit in and not fall out. But the chair wouldn't go. We discovered it needed a key. Long trip through the building to find someone who knew where the key was. Then, now knowing where to look for it, another long trip to get it. Try again. The chair still wouldn't go. But of course! The key also had to be turned at the bottom of the stairs as well as at the top. A trifle awkward if you're in a wheelchair. But then getting into the chair-lift was also awkward, as would be carrying the wheelchair down on your lap - so really this obstacle didn't make it any worse. I just watched the rehearsal, before risking an attempt. Standing is tiring, so I leant on the balcony balustrade and parked my crutches against it. One promptly rotated and slipped between the railings. As I grabbed at it, the other also swivelled and fell through. Fortunately neither speared anyone in the toilet below. (Accidents like this are probably why all crutches now come with rubber tips.) Finally the stair-lift worked. But by now I no longer fancied the acrobatics of getting in to it. Emptying my urine bag into a bowl in the kitchen seemed a lot safer - and, so long as nobody saw it, almost as hygienic.

Lesson to be learnt: the simplest way is usually easiest - even in the kitchen.

Lifts

Fortunately, most public buildings now have proper lifts. These are always big enough for wheelchair and pusher. Frequently, however, they are no bigger. As my feet extend beyond my heels, they also extend beyond wheelchair heel-rests. This means either broken - or at least, bruised - toes, or that the lift door closes on my pusher's bottom. Naturally I prefer the latter option and try to fend myself off the end wall to save my toes. If, as is usually the case, I have crutches over my shoulder, any attempt to save her bottom from the doors means her nose hits my crutches.

Space problems can be even more acute in historic buildings. In one European palace, the lift was artfully fitted into a cupboard. The authentic cupboard door was just wide enough for my wheelchair. Likewise, the cupboard-sized lift was exactly wheelchair size. Unfortunately, the lift was at right-angles to the door, so needed a sharp turn to enter. This may have looked clever on paper, but it demanded even more cleverness of us. How could we turn the wheelchair in so confined a space? The easiest way would be to take me out, fold it, and then carry it in. But where to park me? There was no space to stand. Or was I meant to hang from the ceiling? In any case, aren't wheelchair lifts meant to be for wheelchair *and* occupant?

Ten minutes trial, error and historic-building chips later, and wheelchair and me were in the lift. This wasn't actually so much use. Without my friend, I could go up and down to my heart's content, but never get out. (Fortunately, my heart is easily contented; one journey would suffice. Unfortunately, there's no way the lift could know this.) It took a few more minutes to fit her in too. Fortunately, by now being experienced wheelchair-maneuverers, it took a mere five minutes to get us all out.

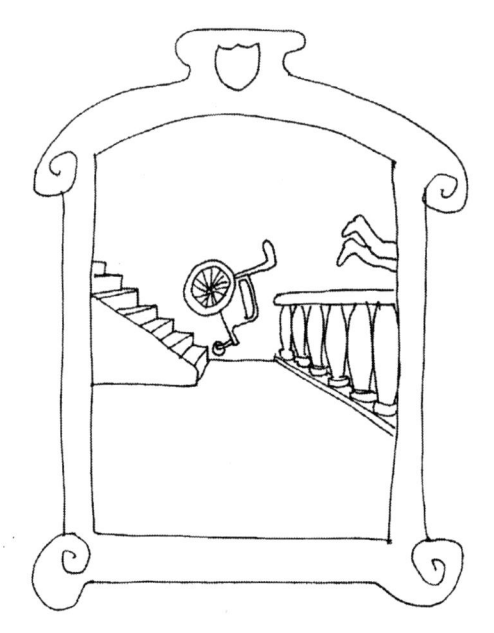

Expect the unexpected in disabled accessible heritage buildings.

Surviving Architecture: non-accessible accessibility

That, however, was the easy bit. As historic buildings don't have cupboards on the ground floor, I needed to climb two sets of steps and one staircase to even get to the lift. The staircase was marble, highly polished. So was its ten inch wide balustrade. My weak hand won't open ten inches, and slips on polished marble. So does my good hand. This made the balustrade, though excellent for sliding down, useless as a hand-grip. (No doubt it was fun for royal children, but not for crippled kings.) Clearly the renovation architect reasoned that if I could negotiate this, the lift would be child's play (just like the banisters). He was right.

Most lifts are easier. Anyway, they're meant to be. All you do is press a button, wait and (eventually) the lift arrives. I then walk at full-speed towards it. Unfortunately, my full-speed is quite slow, so the open door waits for me tantalizingly, then loses patience and shuts just as I get there. So.... Press the button again and wait for the other lift. The one I'm not waiting in front of arrives, so cancelling my call. Door opens and shuts before I get there. Try again...

If I'm lucky, I can get a crutch through the doors to stop them shutting. It never does. If I'm unlucky, the crutch will get caught and go up with the lift, possibly lifting me by the armpit to the ceiling. Hopefully at this point it would shear the crutch and drop me back to the floor. At worst, the door would catch both crutches and take me up five floors - crutch ends inside the lift, me outside. Would this qualify me for air-miles? It is not, however, an advisable method of travel.

Travel inside lifts is preferable to travel outside them.
Unfortunately, lifts don't seem to care which service they provide.

Some lifts have superior technology. One French hotel had a special security system. Just type in your six-figure room code, then the floor you want. By the time I had taken my glasses off, read the code, put glasses back on to free my good hand, the lift had gone off to some other command, and I would have to start all over again. None of this was helped by the French meaning of 'après' - meaning, in this context, 'next', not (as in my dictionary) 'after'. But even when I eventually did everything in the right order, I found the lift thought faster than I moved. Statistics may claim lifts are the safest form of travel. But *I* think they're more dangerous than rock-climbing. Of course, I never climb without a rope.

Lesson to be learnt: don't put too much trust in technological aids. Safety ropes are safer.

Electric Doors

Doors can be heavy to open. This may be awkward, but in a wheelchair it's quite safe - all that happens is that the door reverses me back where I came from. With both sticks and crutches, however, heavy doors are less safe - especially self-closing ones. Some are so heavy - or powerfully sprung - that I must lean against them. This is a precise art. Too much lean and the door swings too far so I fall into the room. Too little lean and the door pushes me backwards so I fall out of the room. Fortunately, there is a technique. I can hold the door open with a well-positioned stick (or crutch). Unfortunately, once I've taken a pace or two, I need to move the crutch. Usually, the pressure of the door has squeezed the rubber ferrule, jamming it. Freeing this is a challenge to balance - and once freed, the door is also freed, so continues its inexorable swing. To complete getting-through-doorway now requires deft footwork, but my feet aren't deft. This means getting through self-closing doors is a doubly precise art. Non-self-closing doors in a wind are even harder. Wind gusts are variable so sometimes I'm leaning too hard, sometimes nowhere near enough. Surviving these is a trebly precise art.

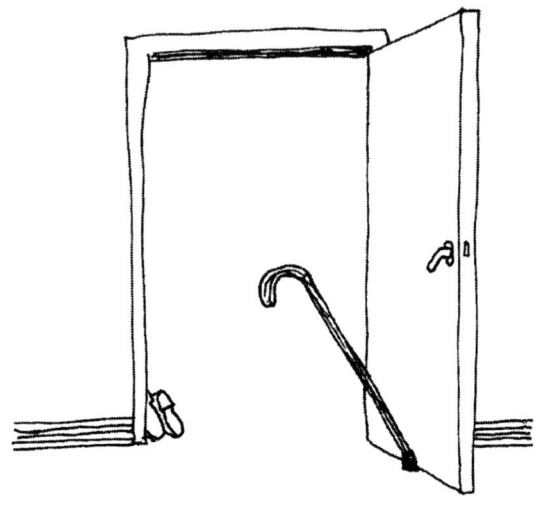

"He went that-a-way."

Surviving Architecture: non-accessible accessibility

Electric doors would be handy here. Or they *should* be handy. The problem is that they are intelligent. Unfortunately, intelligence is only one aspect of personality. It doesn't guarantee friendliness or good will. No doubt some electric doors are friendly. Most aren't. Many have their sensor beam set in front of the door. I approach. Door obligingly opens. I go into doorway. It closes. Not fast, but with determined force. I set my sticks apart and brace myself. Slowly, methodically, and mercilessly, it pushes me over. Even the heaviest (non-electric) hinged doors you can hold open with a well planted stick. Not so electric ones. They're too powerful. Sliding ones are even worse as they push you sideways. Through these, I try to go dead centre. Better to be squeezed from both sides than pushed over. And pushed over I have been, so nowadays I don't dare go through electric doors without help. Electric doors exemplify a major problem of intelligent buildings, namely that often they're not really that intelligent. *They* may think that they are helping - but *I* think that they're just bullies. In short, I don't like intelligent buildings. They have no tolerance of unintelligent people like me.

Lesson to be learnt: intelligence isn't everything; sometimes you need to move fast. Especially with stupid buildings.

Further lesson to be learnt: good will and courtesy are more helpful than intelligence.

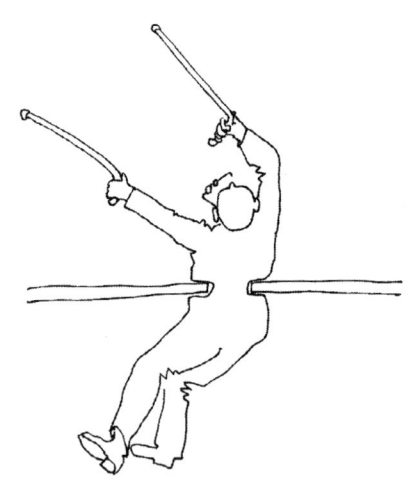

Slim-line electric doors.

12. Getting to Where to Get Cured: Complimentary Therapy Rooms

There is a lot of difference between orthodox and complimentary medicine. Orthodox medicine can't treat me, but its hospitals are fully disabled-accessible. (True: this is only after you've found somewhere to park, walked half-a mile to the door and managed not to get lost in the endless corridors.)

Fortunately, complimentary medicine can treat me, but unfortunately, many therapists work in (almost) inaccessible premises, usually upstairs, often in their homes. Everybody knows their way around their home, so - for them - access isn't a problem. For me, however, it can be. Indeed, the better the therapist, often the less accessible. Possibly the effort of will required to surmount these is part of the cure?

Lesson to be learnt: If you're ill enough to need treatment, don't expect to be able to get there.

For Skenar treatment, I used to go to London. Even though only walking with one stick at that time, public transport was impossible. As I walked too slowly to risk crossing roads to bus-stops, I had to use the Underground. But even outside rush-hour, there were hazards – especially on stairs. I could (reasonably) safely inch down, gripping the handrail, but when I met an old man - obviously as unsteady as me - coming up, what could I do? We both stopped - an impasse. After carefully listening behind (I dared not turn for fear of losing balance), I let go and risked the traverse to the other handrail - hoping I would reach it before the next avalanche of impatient commuters, and also hoping my weak left hand could hold on hard enough. On exposed cliff-face traverses like this, I feel much safer with a rope. Unfortunately, ropes are not in fashion in London. No wonder London is a dangerous place. After this, I realized I would never dare use the underground again. This meant I must travel by taxi - and taxis aren't cheap. But access problems didn't stop there.

Even when arrived, treatment was in a room on the third and a half floor. Fortunately, there was a lift. But the journey wasn't simple. The lift started - as all good lifts should - at the ground floor, and went to the third. But the ground-floor door was locked; it was for goods deliveries only. The front door proper was up some eight steps. There was no handrail, though with iron railings to hold onto, this was no problem. Unfortunately, three quarters of the way up, these stopped at a brick pier. Fortunately, brickwork offers finger-nail purchase in the mortar-joints. Unfortunately, this is not enough for safety. Even when I had reached the top, I still wasn't safe. The landing was swept by the outward-opening door. This door I needed to open with great caution. Doubly great because, at any moment it could burst fully open as someone in a London-hurry rushed out of the building.

Getting to Where to Get Cured: Complimentary Therapy Rooms

Once inside, however, problems still weren't over. First, there was a flight of steps down, fortunately with a handrail. This was necessary to get to ground-floor level, whence all disabled-accessible lifts should start. Then the lift itself. Mostly (two times out of three) it worked. (This meant that one time out of three it didn't, so I had unnecessarily added two extra flights of stairs - one down, one back up - to my journey.) The lift went to the third floor, but not to the half. After that there were only two flights of steps to the half floor.

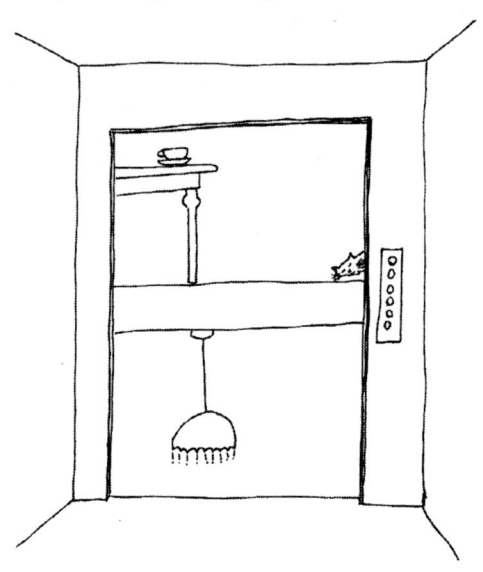

Therapy room on the third-and-a-half floor.

At the end of all this was a couch I couldn't get on. Fortunately, this could be overcome with an upside-down plastic bowl to stand on. Unfortunately, upside-down plastic bowls are of limited use on stairs. This building was clearly designed for disabled accessibility on whole floors, half accessibility on half floors and no accessibility at the entrance. Why, I wonder, did they bother with accessibility at all?

Lesson to be learnt: if you are only half-disabled (namely have one non-working leg) only expect half-accessibility.

Unfortunately, there were still more problems. Being incontinent, I prefer to go to the toilet *before*, rather than (by accident) *during* any therapy session. For not-friendly-cat reasons, I couldn't safely go to the toilet where I was staying and also had a long taxi ride. This meant, immediately on arrival at Skenar-treatment-building, I had to look for a toilet, usually in rather a hurry. The nearest one was on the ground floor. It had no window. As I had more urgent concerns than the view, this was OK if the light was working, but harder if it wasn't. It usually wasn't. Unfortunately, some twelve inches in front of the toilet stool, was a step. In the dark, it was important not to trip over it and fall into the toilet. This was also important in the light, but much easier. (Apparently, this is an occupational hazard for burglars: They like to climb head-first through ever-open bathroom windows. Once through the window, however, there's a major risk of falling head-first down the toilet. Although this makes a serious risk of drowning, burglars find it very hard to get insurance.) The disadvantage with shutting the door was that it made the room dark - hence hard to find my way out. Being locked in a blacked-out toilet is claustrophobic. Being locked in one with a booby-trap is dangerous. Fortunately, I wasn't in a wheelchair in those days. The step would have been perfectly positioned to catapult me head-first into the toilet-pan. And, had I had a pusher with me, there would have been something (someone) else to trip over in the dark. This can't be done silently - there would at least be one squeak. Hence it would be embarrassing when two of us emerged from a darkened toilet. But then, leaving the door open would also be embarrassing.

Lesson to be learnt: look (and remember) before you lock.

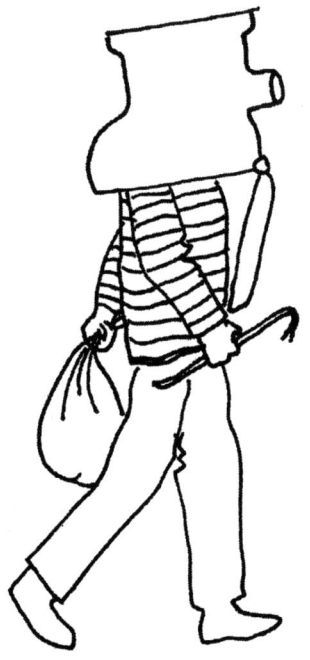

It's easy to recognize novice burglars.

In Wales, the hazards seem humbler - but potentially more lethal. Where I go for acupuncture, the house is single-storey, easy to park near and with a friendly, if clumsy, dog. There is a simple, direct, way in. This, however, involves a flight of steep steps, off which lead other steps at right angles. Instead of a handrail, there is a thorn-bush on the left, and a knee-high stone wall on the right. After trying this once, I now always take the long way. This starts with a sloping

Getting to Where to Get Cured: Complimentary Therapy Rooms

concrete path – easy when dry, but greasy when wet, hence, with crutches, particularly nose-unfriendly. Being near the sea, the view is good, but with view comes exposure to wind. Buffeting gusts of Atlantic gale aren't good for balance - so also not good for noses. Next comes front-door hazard. This is up three steep steps, but first I have to go down one monster one at right angles to them. Additionally, there are various potted plants, Buddha statues and Chinese dragons for good luck. This I need. Indeed, these obstructions don't really help make the steps safer. Moreover, at the top, there isn't a landing: only a storm-sill astride the top step, halving its width. The door itself has so many things behind it, that it only opens half-way. Perhaps that's why there is only a half top-step. Naturally, there's nothing to hold onto except the door - which moves - and its letter-box - which bites me and won't let go. After all this, there's only one place I can plant my crutch: a small mat, slippery as ice.

All this makes the ascent difficult and risky. Much worse - as with all glaciers - is the descent. To add to hazard, friendly-dog usually chooses this moment to be friendly. My therapist however, is resourceful. She made a bridge diagonally across the two flights of steps, so it only sloped 1:4. Being a diagonal, sloping bridge, it also sloped across its width, down to the left. Once my weight was past half-way, therefore, it would tip over to the right. Simple physics made this easy to predict, but simple pathology made it less easy to correct my balance in time. Fortunately, I had her to hold onto. Unfortunately, she is much smaller than me. For additional - or perhaps, the only, 'security', she also provided a safety rope: a child's skipping rope looped over the wind-chimes. As these were only fixed to the wall with two thin screws, I wondered why we needed such strong rope. A piece of wool would have sufficed.

I never had full confidence in this bridge. It was a wardrobe door, about half-an-inch thick, and made of chipboard. Being an architect, I knew that chipboard has no bending strength. Acupuncturists do not need to know this. Clearly - to me - it was only held together by its mahogany-effect paper surfaces. Mahogany-effect paper is slippery, even when dry, which it often wasn't. In addition to paper, one side had a full-size glass mirror. Glass is even slipperier. Fortunately, it was underneath, so *I* was less likely to slip. The *bridge*, however, was more likely to. As it happened, the mirror broke the first time we used this contraption. To avoid further damage to the door, she then rested it on a towel. This may have been good for the mahogany-effect appearance of the door, but it meant the bridge could now slip freely. It did. Slipping bridge, slippery surface, 1:4 slope and 1:6 cross-slope (alternating from side to side) are not a good combination. Nonetheless, I have (to date) survived. I attribute this survival to no longer using the bridge.

Lesson to be learnt: getting to get healed can be dangerous.

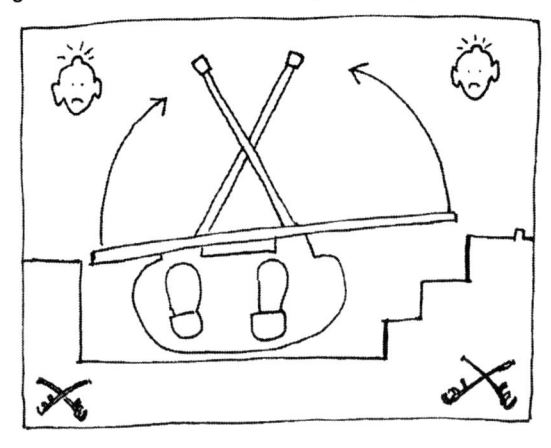

Getting to Where to Get Cured: Complimentary Therapy Rooms

The Pivoting Bridge: this Tarot card signifies the passage from life to death.

Two years prior to this, I used to have acupuncture in a natural health clinic. Like many, it was upstairs, above a health-food shop. (You go to the downstairs shop to stop getting ill; but when you *are* ill, you go upstairs.) Fortunately, in this case, these were narrow stairs. These are much safer than broad ones - if things go wrong, just lean against the wall. At the bend, however, the handrail stopped. Unfortunately, so did one wall; it became full-length curtain. Whereas walls are solid, curtains aren't. Curtain is certainly easier to hold than walls, but not to trust. It pulls down. Pulling down curtains may be fun - two-year-olds love it. But I am not two. And, frankly, I find it less fun at the top of a staircase!

Lesson to be learnt: there's a lot of talk of health and safety, but often the issue is health *or* safety. Which is the more important to choose?

13. Places to stay in; Places not to stay in

Hotels

It's not often I go to hotels, but when I do, I naturally ask for a disabled accessible room. One was arranged for me by the organizers of a conference in Spain. The trip was uneventful till we arrived in Valencia. My assistant put me in my wheelchair and started wheeling me out of the airport. We didn't know where the hotel was, nor what was supposed to happen. (Arrangements in Spain don't seem to be done till the last minute - by which time we were travelling from Wales to London) But everything (or, at least, some things) would probably work out alright - we hoped!

Suddenly, in the crowd, we saw someone holding a sign with my assistant's name on. We made contact and he continued to push me towards the exit. Then a sign with my name on! We stopped, shook hands, then this person took over pushing. Out we went to a taxi-van. I tried to look over my shoulder for my assistant. Not there. The driver hooked up my wheelchair to various straps and winches to pull me aboard. I asked him to look for my assistant. "Si." he beamed and started to winch. I now *ordered* him to look for my assistant. "Si! All OK." and he loaded me on board, shut the door, jumped in and off we drove.

"Which hotel?" I only knew the conference address, something like: "Palacio del Congress", though I could only guess how to pronounce it. Of the hotel, I had no idea; nor of the conference timetable. No hotel address, and now: no assistant, no luggage, no slides or lecture notes - this was not an auspicious start. But this was Spain, so it would probably be alright in the end (I hoped!)

The driver chose a hotel (it seemed to me like a random guess) and asked me if it was right. I had no idea. But it didn't matter what I said. The combination of my weak voice, my position ten feet behind him, traffic noises, the back of his head, his limited English and my (almost) zero Spanish, meant he rarely understood anything I said.

We arrived at this random hotel and he wheeled me up to the reception counter, waved and left. I tried to explain to the counter clerk that I didn't know whether this was the right hotel - wondering what to do if it wasn't. At that moment, my assistant appeared - he had been transported by a second taxi. So, unless we were *both* at the wrong hotel, it was alright in the end. As it should be - this, after all, was Spain.

Our room was luxurious - and spacious. Spacious enough for my assistant to drag his bed into the middle of the room to avoid electro-magnetism from the light switches. Fortunately, he knew enough about electricity to know how important this was. Unfortunately, he did this in the middle of the night.

The bathroom was even more luxurious, even more spacious. It was marble floored and, in the far corner, the toilet had a grab-rail. The shower was easy to walk into (unlike bath-cum-showers which I probably can't get into, certainly can't get out of) and had a fold-down seat. What luxury! All this made it easily disabled accessible.

I rose long before my companion (I hadn't been furniture moving in the middle of the night) and showered. Sitting on the seat, the shower spray bounced off my thighs onto the shower curtain. When I finished, I discovered that this curtain was mounted to hang *outside* the gutter, so directed all water onto the floor. This was awash. I tried it with my crutch. The wet marble was like well-oiled ice. I held onto the shower side. Five feet away was the door handle. Twelve feet away, the toilet grab-rail. Both out of reach. My assistant was asleep (sleeping the sleep of a midnight furniture-mover), and my voice too weak to wake him. The floor was far too hard to risk falling on. I couldn't crawl. If I got down and rolled, I wouldn't be able to get up, so wouldn't be able to reach the door-handle. In any case, rolling through (by now cold) water had limited appeal. What could I do?

I reviewed the situation carefully. First, what about a towel on the floor - would it grip or slip? I poked it with a crutch. It slipped. Was there a route out? I certainly couldn't risk the five feet to the door. So tantalizingly close, but about a foot beyond safely balanced reach.

I crept along the bath edge to the towel rail. Flimsy, but it held. Then the basin lip, then at last the security of the toilet grab rail. But now I was at the opposite end from the door. The walls were also marble. Being luxury standard, the panels fitted closely - no finger-holds here. Fortunately, there were, however, a toilet roll holder and two brass wall-hooks. Unfortunately, when I got to these, they weren't brass, but merely gold-plated plastic and just glued onto the wall. Would they hold? By double good fortune (one per hook), they did. So did the equally flimsy hooks glued to the back of the door. Then - at last - the door-handle! Outside the bathroom, came the safety of the carpet - flooded, but still good friction despite its sogginess. I felt I had finally reached level grass after a hair-raising glacier-traverse!

Lesson to be learnt: 'disabled accessible' means you can get in. It doesn't necessarily mean you can get out.

Further lesson to be learnt: even smooth water can be dangerous.

The most disabled-unfriendly hotel I have yet met was in England. What was called a 'disabled room' certainly didn't feel it. 'Disabling' would have been a better term. The bathroom in particular was a super-slippery-floored death trap. The basin was gracefully modern, hence smooth and lip-less - no hand-hold here. The taps had spherical handles, slippery to grip. When I grasped them tightly for use as hand-holds, they just turned on. The only other possible hold was a fashionably fragile shelf.

Places to stay in; Places not to stay in

To get up from the toilet, there was a limited range of pull up aids, none ideal. There was a toilet-roll holder, but this was only attached by one loose screw. Or I could grasp the electrically heated towel-rail. This boasted a prominent warning-of-burn-if-touched notice - well-founded as I could feel the sizzling heat at some distance. Lastly, there was the door handle, but this was only within reach when the door was open. With handles - on open doors the more so - the trick is not to let go, but - like life - hold on whichever way they swing. Also like life, they eventually stop. Perhaps that's not the most reassuring analogy... Better to say they eventually stop uncontrollably swinging.

Lesson to be learnt: whatever the unanticipated swings, or sideways slides of life, however unappealing the prospects, it's safest to hang on tight.

B&Bs

Guest houses are more friendly than hotels but not necessarily as disabled friendly. At one in Scotland, that my friend/helper and I went to, I was offered a choice of rooms. One had a double bed – very appealing as, unlike my single at home, I could roll over without risk of falling out! But this bed was so high I would be sure to fall off while trying to get onto it. The other room had two single beds put together. This looked ideal. The combined bed would be plenty wide enough for safe rolling. Unfortunately, on landlady-polished floors, two beds like to drift apart. This I discovered by three-quarter falling in between them. I also discovered the bed(s) were so low that I couldn't get *up* off them. Fortunately however, with the rope and handle gadget that I take travelling tied to the window latch, I could pull myself up to uncontrollable-swing level to grab the window-frame (hoping my string wouldn't pull the window shut), then sidle along the wall, grasp the basin taps, turn and sidle along the narrow gap between bed foot and cupboard. Now, at last, something to hold: the cupboard doors. Unfortunately, being sliding doors, these liked to slide. True: it's good to see problems from the other side - but there's also the issue of balance.

Getting to the bed edge and into bed presented similar problems, but in reverse order. As it happens, few things in life are easier backwards. These journeys to and from bed caused many adventures, required many improvisations. Some were ridiculous - but worked. Some were even more ridiculous - and didn't. Between sliding doors, self-propelled beds, self-closing windows and self-opening taps, hardly a handhold could be relied upon; hardly a move produced the intended result. This wasn't dangerous; I could always fall onto the bed - propelling it across the room. But it did cause many laughs. Fortunately - or unfortunately - my friend made tea while I was negotiating Bed-side Obstacle-course. Fortunate, because I enjoy tea. Unfortunate, because hot tea on lap and laughing are not a good combination. I should not, therefore, have been surprised to discover the landlady bent double to check her flower-beds under our window after dark. As we had a jar of live bees for my bee-sting therapy, she got yet another surprise when checking (all part of here landladyish duties) the inside of my cupboard.

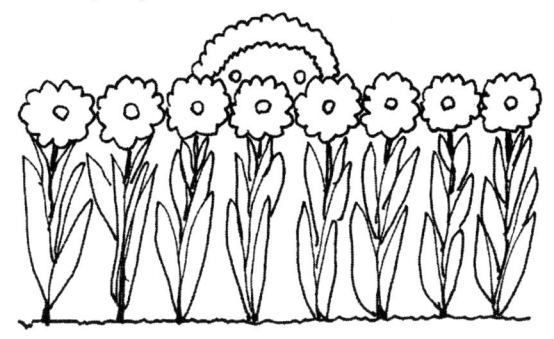

Landlady surveillance.

The bathroom was not set up for disability: instead of a walk-in shower, there was a bath with shower. To keep the shower-spray in – and therefore keep *me* out - this had a glazed screen half way along the edge. This also ensured that there was nothing to hold onto except the basin tap – which promptly turned on, quickly becoming too hot to touch.

Eventually, however, we found a technique. This involved holding onto the toilet hand-rail and leaning forward so my foot could be lifted into the bath. Leaning forward brought my face low down over the toilet. As this couldn't be flushed without robbing cold water, hence scalding (then suddenly freezing) me under the shower, the view was not good.

Guest houses do, however have a more human face than hotels. Although nobody could understand my speech and everyone therefore assumed me half-witted, the landlord - a farmer and dog-show judge - was heard to remark: "He does have intelligent eyes." Obviously, judging dog-shows does come in handy for character assessment.

Lesson to be learnt: B&B usually means Bed and Breakfast (but for dogs: Bed and Bone). Sometimes, however, the Bed can cause problems. (Occasionally even Breakfast and Bones too.)

Places to stay in; Places not to stay in

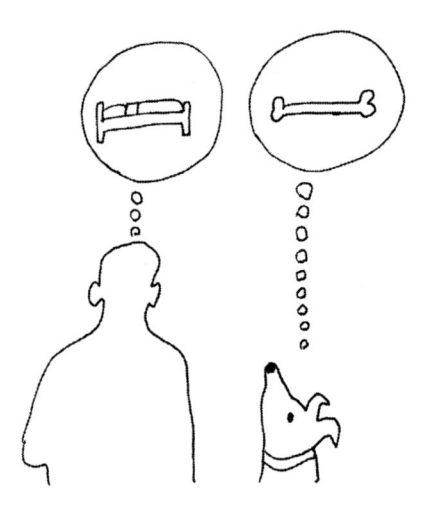

B & B: bed and bone?

Other People's Houses

Not every house is disabled friendly. Indeed, even the best of friends can have unfriendly houses.

One, converted from offices, is upstairs. The stairs present the first challenge to an easy life. Not so much the stairs themselves. These are merely split and ready to break. But the handrail has no topmost support-bracket and the next two are broken, so sways alarmingly. Fortunately, it has never actually come off the wall - yet! This handrail proved an excellent self-development aid as, several times a day, I had to put full trust in: "with love, all things are possible."

Once upstairs, the floor has subtle changes in level. Some slope, some are only about one inch steps, and some move. Fortunately, all these are successfully concealed from view by a loose floor covering. Unfortunately however, the challenge to balance remains.

Like many European houses, every doorway has a three-inch threshold. British visitors usually stub their toes then, a second later, their noses. Generally they do this only once, as the experience is memorable, even if accompanied by a memory-free period. Fortunately, I don't move this fast. But unfortunately, for me these are major obstacles - especially in curtain-covered doorways.

Long curtains are hazardous for sticks and crutches. All too easily these rest on the curtain-tail instead of the floor. As anyone who has had fun - or a fright - sliding on mats knows, loose cloth makes an excellent lubricant. Feet sometimes slip; crutches *always* do. Curtains also like to stick to faces. Hence the combination of a step, lubricant and blindfold made one doorway into a ten-minute obstacle - not ideal on the route to the toilet.

Places to stay in; Places not to stay in

Generally, I beat the doorway, but when the score reached 38 - 1, I thought it time to use a zimmer frame instead of crutches. With curtained doorways, frames are much easier than crutches. Just approach, stop, drape curtain over head, then - as in life - proceed blindly. As long as you are pointed correctly, you'll emerge the other side of the doorway and can undrape the curtain. A good sense of direction helps; so does (blind) faith.

Unfortunately, there were other doorways with steps. One had a tile step. This was slippery and too wide for me to step over. Moreover, it required a right-angled turn. This isn't easy with a wheeled frame. (These, like life-plans, are designed to go forward, straight. Unfortunately, like life, reality is rarely so straightforward.) The frame must, therefore, be lifted and swung at arm's length. In place of blindness, I now had balance difficulties. I know blindness and balance have something to do with justice, but which cause the greater problems in life?

Lesson to be learnt: As in life, you can't always see where you're going. Nor does life always go straight. But you still always get somewhere.

Bathing also proved adventurous. (I anyway never feel safe bathing in unfamiliar waters.) To get into the bath, I would hold the edge with one hand, a wall-mounted handrail with the other, while my friend lifted each leg in turn and swung them in. I would then utilize the bath's slipperiness to spin - hopefully (and usually!) without also sliding - so I could sit on a plank across the bath. But after my shower would come getting out. By sliding the plank along the bath - but hopefully (and usually!) not off its edge - I could reach another handrail to pull myself up on. Now I could hold the washing machine - preferably unplugged so it didn't tingle - while my friend lifted my feet out. This time, however, my feet would be soapy-slippery, and the washing machine offered so little grip that I needed an additional friction hold with my nose (in rock-climbing: a 'nose-hold'). Unfortunately, even when successfully out, my legs would end up crossed and jammed, with me out of balance. I sometimes wondered if cleanliness was worth it!

To some extent, friend's houses can be adapted. Here, we festooned radiators and stair landing with rope. Unfortunately, however tight, rope is always loose enough to swing on. This guaranteed good swinging practice. Fun perhaps, but like abseiling - and perhaps life - there is one golden rule: however hard you hit your knees, scrape your knuckles and face, or otherwise get hurt, *never* let go! Especially, doubly-never, let go at the head of stairs!

In strange - or even normal, but unfamiliar - houses, I myself also have to adapt. Unlike the normal practice of life, this means extreme caution. If the home has good spirit and the friend worth visiting, all this awkwardness – and hazards – is only of secondary concern. By definition, therefore, this makes them manageable.

Places to stay in; Places not to stay in

Lesson to be learnt: Whatever the obstacles, friendship outweighs them.

Friend's toilets are another matter. This is a room it's really nice if I can use. Indeed, disastrous if I can't. Usually, I can get in, but that's only half the story. Getting off the toilet is also important. Although I have only one particular use in mind, it seems that people use toilets for all sorts of things. Dark-room toilets require particular navigational skills. Glass-walled ones are good exercises in pretending not to be embarrassed.

One had a freezer next to the toilet. Indeed the room was either toilet or larder, depending on what you went in there for. It also only had half a floor. The toilet and freezer only just fitted on the wooden half-floor; the rest, one foot lower, was bare concrete. This dual-personality, split-level room meant great agility was required just to get onto the toilet. And even more agility to pull up trousers without falling into it or down the step. Most demanding of all was to get *off* the toilet. For this I had to open the freezer, hold onto its lip and execute cautious and complicated maneuvers. I'm not sure whether this was strictly hygienic, but the alternative was to risk falling, grabbing at the toilet and pulling it off the wall, so severing its connecting pipe. As I couldn't flush it until in a position of safety, this would mean toilet complete with contents all over larder floor. This I judged to be even less hygienic.

Getting off toilets can be a major adventure. Often there's nothing to pull on. Sometimes only a basin inadequately fixed to the wall. Sometimes a radiator. One particular radiator was modern enough to be smooth, smooth enough to be slippery, and on my left. Both my left arm and left pinch-grip are weak. Getting half off the toilet was easy. All I had to do was push up from the seat with my right arm and pull along the radiator with my left. But then my left grip slipped. With shock, all my muscles pull in - the right arm too. This meant it missed the seat and was now positioned directly over the unflushed toilet mouth. It is not funny to plunge your arm down an unflushed toilet. Even less funny if it goes round the bend, where it will surely get jammed as arms are made of straight pieces but toilet bends are, of course, bent. Even less funny again to sit back down on it. I don't want to be taken to hospital with a toilet on my (probably broken, certainly disgusting) arm. What strange perversion would they think I enjoyed doing?

Lesson to be learnt: never lock doors. Rescue is more important than privacy.

Further lesson to be learnt: don't fish down toilets, even if disabled.

Third lesson to be learnt: in mountains, don't go up anything you can't get down. In toilets, don't go (or sit) down on anything you can't get up from (or, if all goes wrong, out of).

Moving around

14. Walking Aids

My first symptoms didn't compromise mobility in any way. Some, like violent leg-quivers when cold, were even entertaining. (After all, I didn't know I was ill, so why not enjoy the slightly ridiculous spectacle?) Six months later, I had developed a discernible limp, though this didn't yet limit life. Soon, however, I found that I couldn't run without tripping. In football games with children, they now always won. (Previously, they often won, but I didn't have the good excuse I now had.) Apart from this, and a weak left-hand so I was no longer an ambidextrous carpenter, my life was unaffected.

When limping began to translate into falls, I began to think a stick might be useful so cut myself an oak-thumb stick. With no rubber ferule, this tended to slip on paving, but on soft ground worked better than a conventional walking-stick. On very soft ground, however, it could stick in and not come out, leaving my momentum to carry me past. This is not ideal. It is the stick equivalent of the Wellington-boot-stuck-in-mud syndrome – equally funny for the observer, equally unfunny for the boot-owner (barefoot - as sock invariably stays in boot) in freezing mud, or for stick-owner (face down in bog).

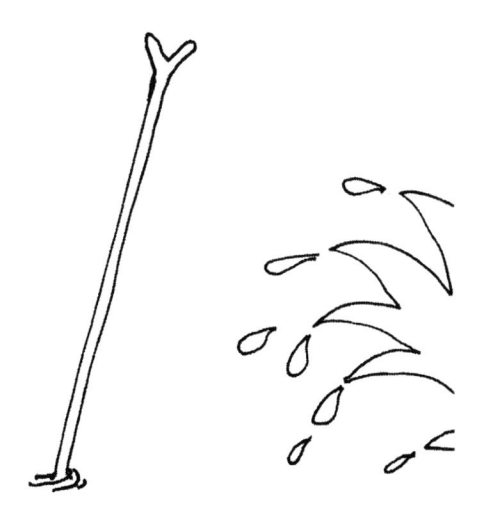

The stick-in-the-mud trick.

The main advantage of a thumb-stick is that it is free to make. The main disadvantage is the happy hiker image. I've nothing against being happy but perhaps others have. Anyway, people tended to be impatient with my slowness; I would routinely be jostled in crowds, and even once had my stick kicked out of the way. With suchlike hazards, I sometimes felt less secure with a stick than without it.

I next progressed to a proper bent-handle stick. This is an invaluable multi-function tool. With its hooked end I could retrieve things from deep under beds, twist it into clothing to lift and carry that from a distant coat-hook to somewhere within reach. Also, if I fell, I could hook it onto furniture to slide myself across the floor to a climb-up point. Additionally, it enabled me to scratch inaccessible parts of my back, pull shoelaces, draw curtains, separate fighting cats. Also a stick extended my zone of offensive action, even from bed, so no alarm-clock within two metres was safe. Unlike cartoons, however, sticks aren't safe for collaring errant children round the neck - even ones who evade washing-up. When one (particularly errant one) tried this on me, it hurt and threatened injury. So better no washing-up than murder (technically: not 'murder', but 'teenagericide'- a lesser offence). Besides all this, sticks are also useful for walking.

Another advantage of walking-sticks is that their hooks make them easy to park. They will hang on counter edges, chair backs, radiators and suchlike. For a hands-free staircase ascent I would hang a stick from my belt or satchel. For descent, however, a stick in this position would snag on the stairs (or, if in front, trip me) so I used to hook it into my shirt collar. This may not *look* very fashionable, or even be too safe, but it is very convenient.

After breaking my rib, I lost confidence in walking and started to use a zimmer-frame. This is stable, but slow. Also, it doesn't hook into shirts, can't collect clothing or naughty children, assassinate alarm-clocks, nor indeed, do much else. In fact, it is a prime example of efficiency: improved performance at the price of versatility. Life being so unpredictable, I often prefer versatility and adaptability to efficiency. Frames also aren't very good on stairs. If you get the balance just right, they're light enough to use like a two-footed stick in one hand (its other two feet are off the step, in the air), leaving the other free to hold the handrail. Unfortunately, I only use a frame because my balance *isn't* good. I am of course grateful to Mr. Zimmer (or was it Mr. Frame?) for inventing it, but as what you can do with it is so limited, I suspect he lacked a sense of humour.

Wheeled frames are even less easy on stairs. These require similar balance skills to mono-cycles. If I could mono-cycle, I doubt I would need a zimmer-frame - anyway not until I fell off the mono-cycle.

Lesson to be learnt: efficiency isn't always such an asset. Versatility is sometimes important – and humour invaluable.

Over time, my legs have become increasingly uncooperative. In fact, they are downright naughty. Spanking doesn't help - another good reason for non-violence - so I now use crutches. These are more stable than sticks. Once on crutches, my fall rate went down from several a month to once every

Walking Aids

two to three months. Like sticks, crutches are easier to walk with going uphill. It may be more work, but there's no risk of runaway acceleration. *Unlike* life - in which it is all too easy - going downhill is harder.

Crutches also look like sticks, though with extensions and arm supports. Unlike sticks, you hold the handles forward. But most people helping me helpfully turn them backward - just like sticks. (Some – the sort of people who *know* they're right - are so helpful, they turn the handles backwards whenever I turn them forwards.) This really would help, were my arms backwards. As they aren't, it doesn't. At this stage, many ask, "Are you alright?" I've learnt it's always wise to think before answering questions. Also, I'm slow to speak and daren't shake my head for fear of losing balance. By the time I answer, they've gone. Some few wait till I can answer "Yes", then ask "Are you sure?" "No" (Of course not. How can anyone be sure about anything in life?)

In most other respects, crutches aren't like sticks. They need special technique on stairs. If you reach forward - up or down - and take a step, you can find yourself suspended from them, feet swinging in the air. This is not good halfway up a stair. It's even worse the whole way up. I therefore demount the crutches from my arms and – as they're not designed for hanging round necks - use them like walking sticks. As I feel much safer gripping a handrail, I hold both crutches in one hand like a two-pronged stick. This works well, but the crutch-heads can become so entwined that they won't separate at the top of the stairs. This is not a good place to let go of the handrail and wrestle with recalcitrant arm-grips.

Sitting down with crutches requires special technique. After getting myself perfectly aligned, I can reach forward with the crutches for counter-balance, bend my knees slowly - for muscle exercise - and sink into chair. Usually the last bit of the descent isn't a controlled sink, but an uncontrolled fall. As long as I don't break the chair, hit my head or funny-bone, this is (more or less) OK, but not very graceful. Likewise, turning is slow, and needs great care. So laborious is it, I feel like a ship turning in harbour - and, like a ship, if I do it wrong I bump the chair - or quay-side - with potentially damaging consequences. Unlike a ship - which damages the quay - I don't hurt the chair, only myself.

In contrast to sticks, crutches are awkward in cars. Sticks are satisfying to throw across to the passenger seat. Crutches bounce back across my seat so I can't get in. Again, unlike sticks, crutches are too long and hinge-topped to press down the passenger door lock. This means that locking by key adds ten minutes - unless I drop the key: then add at least another half-hour.

Like sticks, crutches don't like wind. More exactly, *I* don't. Being unstable, wind can easily blow me over. Even if it doesn't, gusts can blow a crutch away from where I thought I was putting it. This may sound less serious but it has the same result. Also wind brings rain; and the wetter the paving the more likely

Walking Aids

that crutches slip - again, the same result. Poor nose! For safety, therefore, I like to walk along building edges. This way I can plant my crutches where friction from the wall keeps them from slipping. Unfortunately however, walls deflect wind so it shears along them with double the force. Double force wind is cold, but, fortunately, bulky clothes can keep you warm. Unfortunately, with bulky clothes you can easily fly. Flying with crutches isn't easy to control, nor is it very aerodynamic, so a crash landing is likely. Indeed – as all ascents are followed by descents - this is actually preferable to remaining airborne.

Wind makes some places more crutch-dangerous than others. Amongst the worst are motorway service stations. With lots of space allowed for cars, there's high wind-risk. (The same can be said for their food, but that's another issue.) Tall buildings are even worse. These can cause savage down-draught gusts, and - more alarmingly - up-draughts too. Fortunately - not being very keen on flying - I don't live near any. Hospital car parks are also bad places for wind. In one gale, I had to claw my way along a line of ambulances, holding on to whatever I could, and waiting for lulls to cross the small gaps between them. Unfortunately, my journey ended with the hospital building, its corner concentrating the wind to treble force. Fortunately, of all places to have an accident, hospitals are the most convenient - not that I found that particularly confidence-building. Doubly fortunately, I didn't. Fortunately again, both wind and flying can be avoided. As in life, there's always a final alternative: don't go out.

Lesson to be learnt: life is safer near something secure.

Further lesson to be learnt: bigger can be unfriendlier.

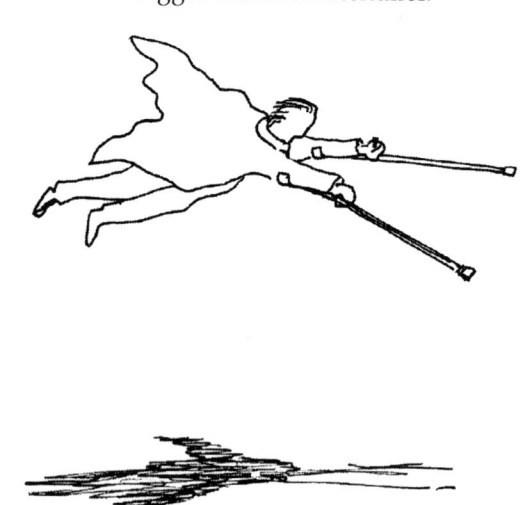

Crutches aren't really designed for flying.

Walking Aids

This is not the only crutch-wind issue. Aluminium crutches are made in two telescoping parts with a spring-loaded stud and adjustment holes. This makes them easy to adjust for length, but in heavy rain they can fill with water. They then slurp rudely when I walk and spill untidily over the carpet when lain (or fallen) down. Wind, however, has less predictable consequences. The holes play Aeolian flute tunes.

Initially I found these ethereal noises disquieting, but now I know that by altering alignment, I can influence the tune. Though crutches have a limited musical range, they can be used to applaud music by others. My hands move too slowly to clap, so I bang my crutches together. On one occasion, somebody behind me said "That is crutch clap." This sounds a painful and contagious condition, but actually using crutches like this is neither painful, nor need affect anyone else.

One other (small) problem with crutches is moles. Moles though small, are no problem themselves. Their holes, however, are. When I plant a crutch over a mole-mound, it can sink deep into the hole. With one crutch six inches shorter than the other, I immediately list, and - if not quickly caught - will capsize.

Lesson to be learnt: sometimes the little things in life have big consequences.

The main disadvantage of crutches is that I can't carry anything. This, of course, isn't necessarily a disadvantage. In the past, the rich never carried anything - their servants did. In my case, however, family members occasionally get fed up with being servants, so luxury is intermittent. Also I'm not rich.

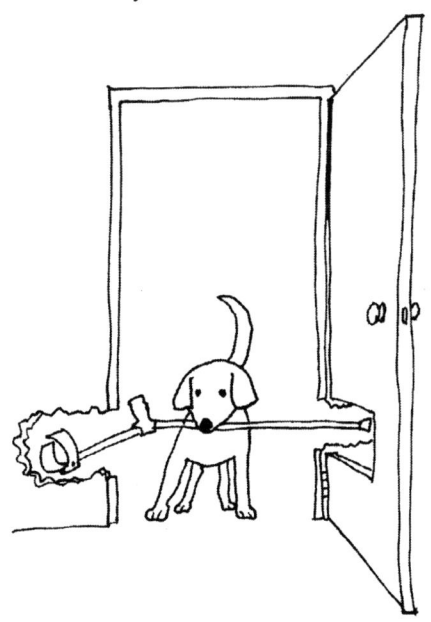

How to retrieve dropped crutches?
Solution 1: train-a-dog (It may be necessary to modify doorways).

Walking Aids

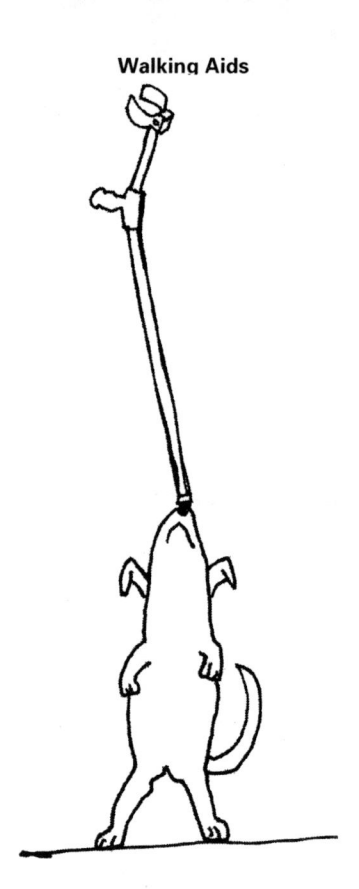

Solution 2: train-a-performing-dog.

Crutches are hard to park, so even if I could carry things, I couldn't collect them. Like sticks, crutches have handles, but these aren't hooked so don't grip on furniture. Moreover, their balance is visually misleading, so even after three years experience I lean them one way only to see them roll over and slide to the (inaccessible) floor. Nor can you pick up things with them. The arm-grip top can indeed hook things, but being pin-hinged, can't hold them.

Not being able to carry things can make life difficult. True, if the things are small enough, I can hold both thing and crutch-handle in the same hand. But I can only *grip* one. Which is more important: thing or safety? Possessions or life? To overcome this dilemma I have a trolley. On this, I can put any items essential to survival - like a cup of tea - or anything else I wish to move around. It is designed to be easily pushed, so runs delightfully freely. I am unsteady on my feet but fortunately, if I feel I'm falling forward, I can lean on the trolley. Or if I'm falling backwards, I can pull on it. Unfortunately, the trolley does not have brakes. This means that if I lean forward, it accelerates and I have to run, as best I can, wherever it decides to go. If I pull back, it will come too, riding up onto my toes so I can't step backwards. A fall is now inevitable.

Walking Aids

So, shortly afterwards, are the contents of the trolley as I unavoidably pull it over on top of me. Despite the importance of tea, I prefer, therefore, not to relinquish crutches.

Using crutches, there is no way I can hold the trolley, so I push it in the direction I wish it to go. My floor isn't level; indeed, the passage slopes downhill. This means that the trolley can choose whichever way *it* wants to go. Fortunately, it has four wheels, which gives it stability. Unfortunately, each wheel is independently pivoting. This means that, like life, the smoother - or stronger, or more bossy, or most strong-willed, or just most obstinately rigid - wheel takes charge. As my room has four walls, but only one me, it's much more likely to visit a wall than come to me. This does not help tea stay in cup. Indeed, it's one reason why I consider tea so essential to life: it rarely arrives.

Lesson to be learnt: it's commonly said, that at the end of life's journey you can't take possessions with you. I believe this. In my experience, at the end of *any* journey, I can't even take tea.

Additional lesson to be learnt: If you want something enough, you'll almost always get it – but invariably in a condition that makes you wish you had never wanted it.

Final lesson to be learnt: once you set out, you never know where you will end up.

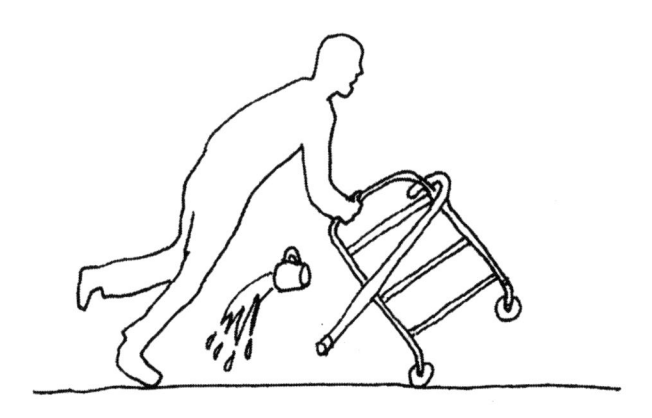

Warning: No horn or brakes means trolleys have no tea.

Multi-aid maths

Walking-aids are useful. With them, I can measure my deterioration rate. How long was I on sticks? How long have I now been on crutches? What about sometimes using a frame? A wheelchair? Does that count as still being on crutches? Can I calculate how long till I'll be bed-bound, unable to move? (Let's not go there.) More practically, how will I manage the stairway to heaven by wheelchair? Or does this mean the only disabled route is downhill?

15. Wheelchairs

Wheelchairs look harmless, but you can never be sure. Mine comes with a safety warning. In big letters this reads: **'WARNING DO NOT blur blur blur blur** ...'. This looks deadly serious, perhaps even a matter of life and death, so whenever I use it I wonder if I am doing, or not doing, whatever 'blur' is.

Despite such latent threats, wheelchairs are fun. I have a 'Little Zipper'. It doesn't zip and though not large isn't particularly small, so makes me wonder how big a 'Big Zipper' is. Nor is it particularly fast, so how slow is a 'Big Plodder'?

Wheelchairs are (reasonably) safe. They don't (normally) fall to pieces on rough ground; their brakes (usually) work on level ground. So long as they've been opened up properly and correctly secured, they don't usually fold. (It is actually rather important that they don't, as folding means passenger sandwich.) The main problem with wheelchairs, however, is their drivers.

Somewhat surprisingly, wheelchairs come with seat-belts. You wouldn't think they would go fast enough to need them. This would be a mistake. Normally, the seat-belts just dangle down and get caught in the wheels. But some drivers need seat-belts. (That is: the passenger needs the belt to survive; the driver needs it as protection against law-suit.)

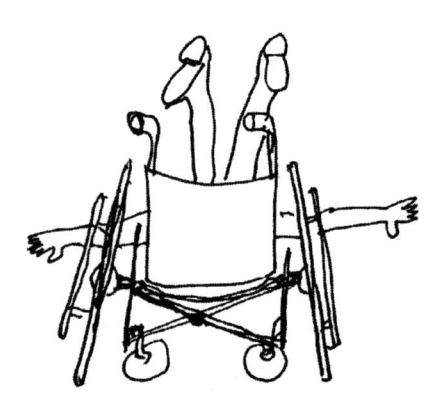

It is recommended to fasten seat-belts before take-off.

One driver helped me out of a car into my wheelchair parked on a steep hill. No brakes on, but, on the rough ground, the wheelchair stood still, politely patient. It changed its mind, however, the moment I sat heavily into it. Obviously wheelchairs are easily upset. Unfortunately, I have only one good hand, so can only reach one brake. Fortunately, I could operate it before the wheelchair accelerated downhill, so it only pivoted in a half-circle. We then set off. My pusher regarded the rough ground as an obstacle to overcome. I kept my mouth shut. If I had opened it to urge caution, I would have bitten my tongue at

Wheelchairs

each bump. At the first pause, I strapped in. Just as well! We approached a kerb. This would be hard to get over. But, with sufficient determination, there's always a way! *One* way is to take a run at obstacles and jump them. I opened my mouth to speak, then shut it to save my tongue. We took the run. The wheelchair stopped dead. Had I false teeth, these would have flown out and impaled themselves in the fence ahead. Even my own teeth wanted to!

Kerbs aren't the only dead-stoppers. Soft sand does it too. It's safer for false teeth - they're less likely to break on the soft ground, but could bite an innocent sunbather. Flying teeth, however, can spear through the surface and get lost - until, perhaps months later, someone sits on them. Imagine the shock of being bitten by the sand!

Lesson to be learnt: wheelchairs don't go with false-teeth.

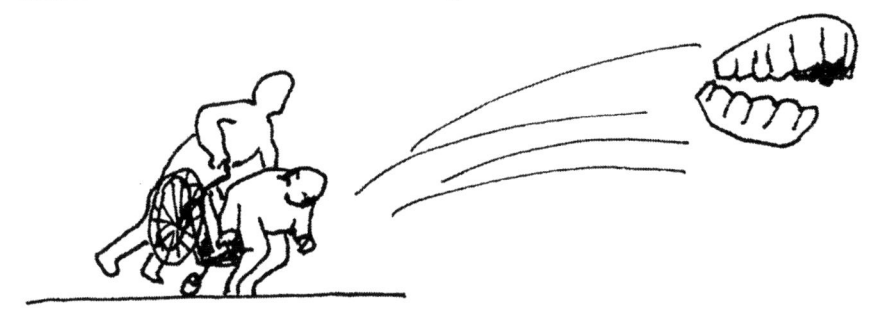

Dental advice: never attack obstructions head-on.

Wheelchairs make you very aware of texture. Cobbles, for instance, give a staccato rattling (also not teeth-friendly). Soft grass is bogging down. Gravel is alright to be pushed on, but not good for self-propulsion. When sitting at an outdoor café table, I tried to turn for a different view, but all I could do was make two clouds of dust. One in front of the right wheel; one behind the left one. The wheelchair remained where it was. All that changed was the dust scum settling on my coffee.

Going to town means steep tilts up pavement kerbs, then immediate right-angled pivots to avoid nose squashed on shop window. Narrow pavements where two wheels are in the gutter, two up on the kerb, don't feel very secure. It feels like I'm about to fall out - and fall roadwards at that! I am. Moreover, these pavements are only narrow because there's not enough roadspace, so traffic comes awfully close to my overhanging head!

One major advantage of wheelchairs in town is that they're good for begging. Waiting outside a shop in Prague, a stranger suddenly offered me money. Although touched, I was too surprised to thank him. I hadn't realized I look *that* pathetic. Only later did I discover that what he offered me was the exact coin I would need for a public toilet. Obviously I must have looked like I needed the toilet.

Wheelchairs

I also have an electric chair. It's called the "Harrier" and can indeed harry people, even though only at a modest 4 mph. I'm told I shouldn't call it an electric chair - the health-outcome associations are wrong.

It may not be fast, but it *is* strong. In children's hands it can push fragile antique furniture around the room, crash its frame-busting way through doorways it isn't properly aligned for, and force low lying obstructions up the wall. Children love it; sleeping dogs don't.

Lesson to be learnt: electric chairs may be a good solution to naughty children, but don't help dogs sleep.

The Harrier is an 'indoor-outdoor' wheelchair. Whatever damage I do with it indoors is my problem, but outdoors, I (in control of it - or not) am a potential risk to the public. Before I could be allowed one, I had, therefore, to take a driving test. There were several parts to this test. Firstly vision. I can see - so that was OK. More demanding was peripheral vision. The tester stood behind me, spread his hands in front of both sides of my head and wriggled his fingers. Could I see them? Of course I could. He then gradually withdrew his hands, asking me to tell him when they disappeared. I am slow to speak, so by the time I had said "Now!" they were a long way back. I passed this test.

Next came the indoor driving test. Operating an electric chair couldn't be simpler - just move a knob in the direction you wish to go. Two things, however, can go wrong. If the chair is switched on when sit down in it, you're sure to knock the knob - and off goes the chair with you half in it, in who knows what direction. (This is one reason why you should never leave them switched on. The second reason is that the cat may jump onto the chair, striking the knob; the third is that if a burglar sits in it for tea-break, he can do lots of damage, so face a more serious charge in court. Burgling may be illegal, but this - like life - is *unfair*.) The other problem is that I learnt to drive with a hand-throttle on a tractor. To stop a tractor, you push the throttle lever forwards while stamping on the brake (and later, the clutch). On an electric chair, stamping has no effect, but pushing the knob has. It immediately accelerates you exactly towards whatever you are trying not to hit. I therefore suffered from the same mis-learning that my son did, when starting to drive. He had learnt from computer games that to turn - even slightly - you must wrench the steering wheel as far as it can go. When he drove me in a real car, this did not reinforce my sense of security. Fortunately, in my case, I managed to make it look as though I had actually intended everything the self-willed electric chair did - so passed the test.

Now, the outdoor test. Here, I had to drive along a pavement (sidewalk), then cross the road to the other pavement. Going down from pavement to road is easy. Crossing the road is just a matter of not hitting any cars. (This would be bad, as electric chairs aren't normally insured to pay for damage to cars -

Wheelchairs

and I myself probably wouldn't be in a state to, after hitting one.) Mounting kerbs, however, needs technique.

First, you eye the kerb: is it within the five inch climbing limit? (Actually, I forgot to say, *first*, you look right and left for traffic. It is inadvisable to forget this too often.) Then you charge at full speed. With luck, the electric chair gets up onto the pavement. (Without luck, you do - but without the chair.) Instantly, you must decelerate by pulling the knob back - but not too far back or you will reverse back into the road - then turn along the pavement. In the hospital car-park, with few cars, no pedestrians and wide pavements, this wasn't *too* hard. In town, dodging traffic, pedestrians and unpredictable children and dogs, this would be less easy. Moreover, most pavements anywhere near where I live are narrower than the chair is long. This makes turning-on-the-spot skill essential for nose-protection.

Having (only just) passed this test, I now became eligible for my very own electric chair. When, eight months later, it arrived, the first instruction in its accompanying booklet told me that it was not legal to drive it on the road. So much for road-tests! Obviously it must be an exclusively off-road vehicle. Too heavy for even two men to lift into a car, it was presumably designed for off-roading at home. I tried it out, therefore, on my lane. Within a few yards, its small wheels bogged down in mud and potholes. My son pushed it out and I walked home with crutches.

Lesson to be learnt: sometimes walking is quicker.

Further lesson to be learnt: not everything that you have to learn, can you always use.

Final lesson to be learnt: electric chairs aren't *always* fun.

16. Disabled-unfriendly Cities

Some cities are wonderful to walk around. But less fun in a wheelchair. Edinburgh, for example, used to be one of my walking favourites. It has characterful cobbled streets (in a wheelchair, however, these equal broken teeth), intriguing passages that end dramatically in cliff-top stairs (equals: dead-end - or, with speed descent - dead on arrival).

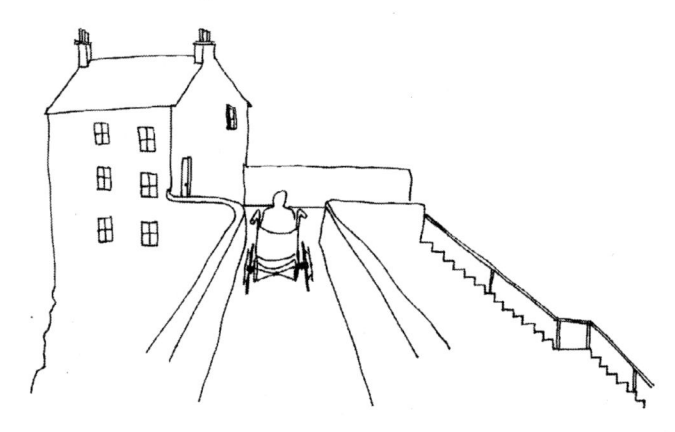

Dead end or Dead at end?

Despite dental bills, cobbles look quaint. Unfortunately, however, they tend to trap the wheelchair's little front wheels, turning them in unpredictable directions. If in the same direction, this means sudden swerves, which on a steep street can bring capsize. If in opposite directions, this means dead stop, usually in the path of an on-coming taxi - whose driver KNOWS we will get out of the way.

Another problem with cobbled streets is that the vibration shakes my footrests loose. They then do the splits, taking my feet with them. Fortunately, this is easy to remedy with string – just tie them together. Unfortunately, there isn't always string to hand. So…. improvisations to the rescue (again). All I need do is tie my shoelaces together. Problem solved! If, however, we come to somewhere where I need to walk, this is no longer easy.

Lesson to be learnt: the simplest way of solving one problem can create others.

Old-town Edinburgh kerbs are eight inch - totally uncrossable by wheelchair. (These would be easier to step over, were my feet not tied.) Fortunately, however, there are concrete ramps at street corners. These, being afterthoughts, slope at forty-five degrees, so wheelchairs prefer to stop dead rather than mount them. If I'm not strapped in, this provides a quick, but uncomfortable, way onto the pavement. Going down, invariably the wheels engage in the cobble patterns so the wheelchair both turns *and* stops. As it does this when sloping forward at forty-five degrees, this provides an even quicker way to the gutter where I can pretend to be drunk. I learnt from a horse that didn't like to jump streams that the combination of forward slope, swerve and sudden stop is a very effective way of dispensing with rider. It seems my wheelchair has read the same textbook.

Edinburgh also has steeply sloping streets. As a passenger, these are quite comfortable - going uphill. I can sit back comfortably, no risk of falling forward. Sometimes, however, I get the feeling we're going slower and slower, while the sound of breathing behind becomes louder and conversation ceases entirely. It seems we stop more often - and here I'm concerned that the brakes hold, which they seem reluctant to do. Reversing at speed is not my idea of fun.

Everybody says going downhill is easier. ("It's all downhill and the wind's behind yer" as my swimming instructor used to say.) Neither has been my experience. I was - and still am - convinced the pool was level; and descending steep streets isn't good for hair colour - unless you like white.

One hill in particular is my least favourite: a long, curving, main-road. It starts innocuously enough, parallel to the contours, but then swings till it points directly down the slope. Fortunately we started on the downhill side. As motorists know, centrifugal force pushes a speeding car outwards on a bend. Traffic engineers, therefore, camber roads so the insides of bends are lower than the outsides. Meticulous traffic engineers also include the pavements. Unfortunately, wheelchairs are not designed to travel at these speeds. Being (mercifully!!) slower, they drift sideways down the cross-slope. Had we been on the outside of the bend, this would have meant a relentless, totally unstoppable, slide towards the curb. This was a two-step curb (each step eight inches high). By guaranteeing good separation of pedestrians from traffic, this made it extra safe - for them. Sixteen inches, however, would be enough to roll a wheelchair. Fortunately I was strapped in, so in no danger of falling out. I would merely have rolled across two bus-lanes and assorted other traffic and hope to finish up upside-down. (The right way up would mean wheels down, hence speed descent of the street. As I would be on the wrong side of the road, in an unlicensed vehicle, and by now without glasses, nor with any semblance of control, this would be illegal.) Doubly fortunate we were on the other side.

I was aware of my pusher pulling, her footsteps increasing in speed and making sliding noises. Could she hold me? I began to regret eating breakfast - that extra weight could be the last straw. Could I help? I considered the options: Holding onto the railings would check, probably stop, us - but almost certainly at the price of a broken arm. Arms are useful, not least for walking with crutches, so perhaps this wouldn't be a good idea. Or I could reach forward with my crutches and use them to stop us. This, however, would have a pole-vault effect.

Disabled-unfriendly Cities

As I was strapped in, this would mean pole-vaulting with a wheelchair. As far as I know, even professionals don't do it like that. Indeed, I doubt it is safe. Furthermore, my pusher (now puller) was hanging on to the handles for grim death (or, if we were lucky, dear life) so all three of us (me, wheelchair and her) would have pole vaulted. As two of us (me and wheelchair) would have landed on her, and as she was my friend, I didn't think this would be a very nice thing to do.

By great good fortune, a bus-stop swung into view. I pointed with my crutches. (Conversation was impossible at this speed.) The queue of people would make a perfect soft braking system. I aligned my crutches across the arm-rests to spread our impact over as many bodies as possible - better to bruise many than run over one. This would be fairer for them, and safer for me. What if I aimed at one but missed? (Moreover, as wheelchairs' narrow wheels make deep ruts in anything soft, and I also had a running puller behind to literally run-over the selected unfortunate, there would be less compensation repercussions.) By even greater good fortune, the slope suddenly eased and my friend was able to regain control.

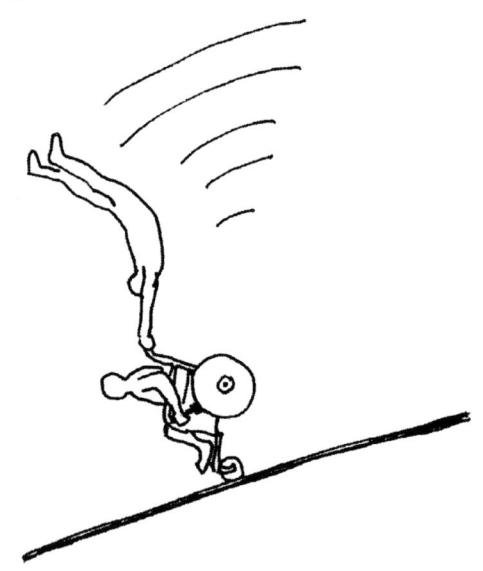

On steep slopes, braking isn't always the safest way to stop.

Lesson to be learnt: always aim at bus stops.

Other lesson to be learnt: always trust in guardian angles.

Edinburgh may not have been built for wheelchairs, but at least it was made for pedestrians. Not so Californian cities. In one I used to work in, pedestrians could only (legally) cross main roads at traffic lights. For several minutes, the light would spell "DON'T WALK", then it would change to "WALK". As it changed back to "DON'T WALK" when I had only crossed three out of ten lanes,

Disabled-unfriendly Cities

what it actually meant was "RUN". Furthermore, as vehicles turning right are allowed through red lights and their drivers know there wouldn't be any pedestrians (who could be that stupid?), pick-up trucks - and larger - would hurtle towards me at 45 mph.

Once I started to limp, and so couldn't run, I stopped ever venturing to the other side of the road. For anyone with even slight walking (or sight) disabilities, the signs should read: "DON'T WALK" and "DIE". The roads may be wheelchair-friendly, smooth and level and the three-inch curbs easily negotiable, but don't be fooled.

Lesson to be learnt: the smoothest roads lead to twenty-two-wheeled trucks. Wasn't there a biblical warning about easy roads? Perhaps it's something to do with all life, not just wheelchairs?

Few British towns are really wheelchair friendly. Most have bits built before cars, which need therefore to be brought up to at least nineteenth century standards. It is well-known that steam gives way to sail - though it's a rash sailor who puts it to the test with a supertanker, which takes two miles to respond to helm or engine reverse. The rule of the road is more pragmatic: foot gives way to car, car gives way to truck. This means roads must be wide, but pavements may be narrow. Most, though unfortunately not all, are wide enough for a wheelchair. But some streets are lit at night. This can mean pavements not wide enough for street-lamp *and* wheelchair. Fortunately, this only happens every forty yards or so. But, however strong-armed or electric-powered, what should the intrepid wheelchairist do? No space to turn means going sideways off the curb, two wheels on pavement, two on road. Result: nose on road. Reversing when you can't turn round requires a high degree of optimistic faith; you put yourself in God's hands. This makes urban wheelchairing a bit like life: Unexpected dead ends in front. Juggernaughts - or, at least, tarmac nose - to the side. Or a long, blind journey trusting in God. This last option is the one I would choose - and so far, I'm enjoying it.

17. Public Toilets: Getting In, Getting Out, and Getting to Use Them

Getting to Toilets

Disability legislation requires public buildings to provide disabled toilets. It doesn't require these to actually *be* accessible. Consequently, some places, like stations, street toilets and motorway 'service' (meaning: take money, don't serve) stations, routinely lock disabled toilets. Presumably disabled people inject more heroin than 'normal' people. Or perhaps heroin injectors are - or become - more disabled? Fortunately, these toilets are usually placed conveniently close to the disabled parking bay - though often this is occupied by a very un-disabled-looking car. Unfortunately, locked toilets are of limited use. Easy as it (usually) is to get to the toilet, getting the key is less easy. There may be steps. Or I may have to go through the restaurant to the cashier at the till. If nothing else, it means a long walk. At my speed, what was originally mildly urgent, now becomes a crisis.

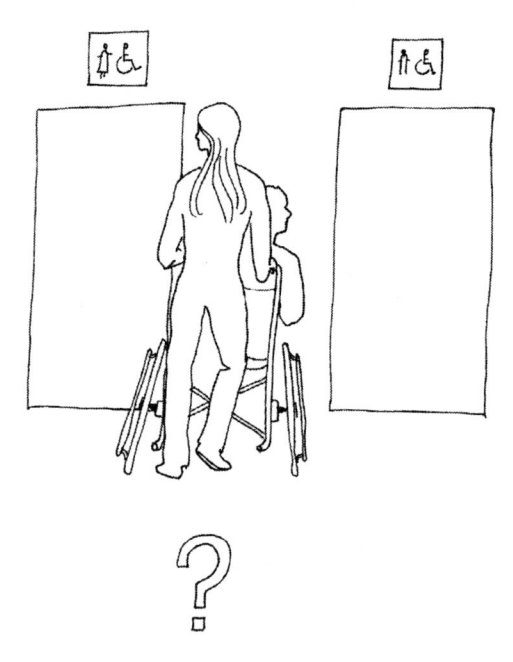

American airports provide twice as many disabled toilets: at each point, one for men, one for women. But which one for us?

In restaurants, however, I must run the gauntlet of other people's legs tripping over the crutches. People get very rude about being tripped, but when they look for someone to shout at, they don't find me - I'm already below eye level, on the floor, hoping that I'm not just about to be buried by the contents of their lunch tray.

Public Toilets: Getting In, Getting Out, and Getting to Use Them

There are also inanimate dangers like spilled chips, greasy floors and plastic or paper litter on which crutches slide even faster than on small mats on polished floors. Transparent plastic sweet papers combine near invisibility with lethal slipperiness.

Lesson to be learnt: beware the dangers of fast-food - especially underfoot.

It's tempting just to use the 'ordinary' toilet. At least, it would be tempting if I hadn't tried this before. What may seem a normal - namely, only slightly slippery - floor is homicidal once you use crutches for stability. One place I do not want to fall, is into a public urinal. (True: many are perfectly shaped for heads, complete with narrower, guillotine-block shaped neck-rests. This, however, does nothing to increase their appeal.) For safety therefore, I walk round the edge of the room, my crutches against the wall. But as, to prevent people looking in, the wall takes many turns, this is a long journey. Unreasonably long, for who on earth would want to look in? Personally, I can't wait to get out!

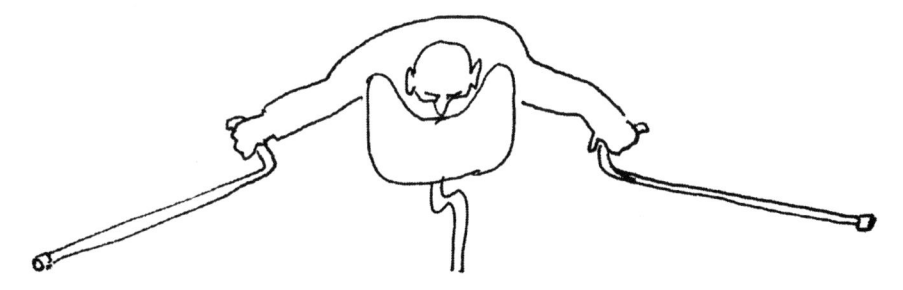

Some urinals are considerately shaped for neck comfort.

To be really safe, I don't use public urinals any more. I would rather use a flower-bed - and as I now wear a bag instead of nappies, this is often the only place I can empty it. This is illegal: it's called 'committing a public nuisance'. But if I don't commit a public nuisance, my bag will burst and then I will commit a private nuisance, with the ensuing overflow making a public one. Fortunately, architects always think of everything: public buildings always have toilets. I'm meant to use them. Even after getting to them, however, they're rarely problem-free. I need to lift my bag-leg to urinal or toilet-seat height. I can't. It needs a hand to lift it. This means I must stand on one leg, holding on with one hand. Two-point support is not very stable - with crutches, I never have less than three. And this would be a bad place to fall. Moreover, in non-disabled toilets, the only thing at the right level to hold onto is the toilet or urinal rim. Now I need to open the bag tap. As I don't want my foot to fall into the toilet, I can't let go, so the tap needs another hand. True: I'm glad not to hold the toilet rim, but I am now standing on one leg, holding on to nothing. Ballerinas do this all the time - and even pirouette. But I am not a ballerina - and the last thing

Public Toilets: Getting In, Getting Out, and Getting to Use Them

I want to do here is pirouette. This is why I prefer flower-beds. If sufficiently dilute, what I have to offer is good for them. It's certainly good for me to give it away. Anyway flower-beds also look nicer. Every public building should have flowers as well as toilets.

Lesson to be learnt: giving can benefit both parties. If you look far enough afield (or a-flower-bed) you can usually find a symbiotic solution.

Baser lesson to be learnt: I must learn to be toilet-wise as well as street-wise.

Fortunately, some toilets are easy to get into - all you need is to know *how*. One old railway-station had been disabled-accessiblized with lifts. One storey below the platforms was the concourse (level -1). Here (almost) were the toilets. 'Almost' because, although the signs were here, they were in fact a few steps further down. Only a short flight, but unfortunately, in a wheelchair, they might as well be across an ocean. Fortunately, however, the lift also went to level -2. At least, there was a -2 button. But it wouldn't go. Press again. No response. Multi-press in various dance rhythms. Eventually the doors did close. But then the lift went *up*! Someone above must have called us. Once higher-being had completed his journey, we tried again. Still no luck. This was getting urgent. In desperation, I tried the -3 button - perhaps the stairs from here might be shorter. Jubilation (possibly misplaced) - it *would* agree to go to -3! When the doors opened, however, level -3 was a forbidding prospect. A gloomy, lifeless corridor, not even relieved by a toilet sign; deathly cold - perhaps it led to the morgue? It also smelt of drains - to which it presumably was near, possibly even connected. Other than retreat back into the lift, there was only one way we could possibly go. Smell confirmed this was the right way. Sure enough, round two corners, there were the toilets, reassuringly (or disquietingly) empty but for their attendant. But why -3 for two floors down? Is it because, asked to pick a number, most people choose 3? (Few, however choose -3.) Or does a three-floor lift have higher status than a two-floor one? (Even if it goes down - not up - and to particularly low-appeal toilets?)

Lesson to be learnt: In navigation, sometimes it's best to follow your nose.

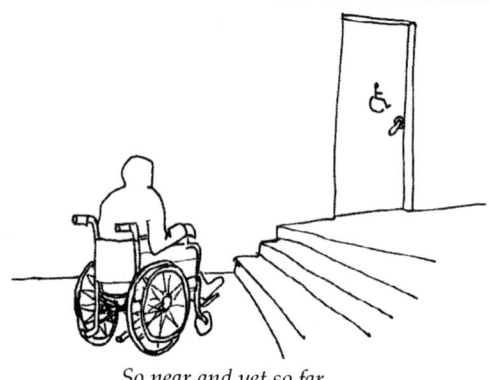

So near and yet so far.

Public Toilets: Getting In, Getting Out, and Getting to Use Them

Getting into Toilets

Not uncommonly, all toilets in a building open off a single passage. First, there is a door to keep them out of public view, and act as a smell and embarrassing-sound barrier. Regulations require this passage to be wide enough for a wheelchair. But sometimes it's not much wider and the disabled toilet is at the passage end. Fortunately, you can turn a wheelchair in its length if it's positioned just right. Unfortunately, it rarely is. It therefore requires careful back and forward maneuvers to successfully turn. These are less easy when being pressed sideways by the self-closing door. They are even less easy when one arm is pinioned against the wheelchair by the very determined door, and only one is free to rotate only one wheel. Turning one wheel but not the other is good for cornering - but I'm not yet positioned to go *round* the corner, only *into* it.

Fortunately, in the worst of such passages (in the glossiest of plush new buildings) I had a helper. I couldn't have done without her. But, space being limited, the door had to close before the wheelchair could turn. This left her on one side of the door, unable to open it because of me on the other side. All things can be resolved in the end - and eventually were - but bladders are impatient; they won't wait for ever.

Lesson to be learnt: self-control can save much embarrassment.

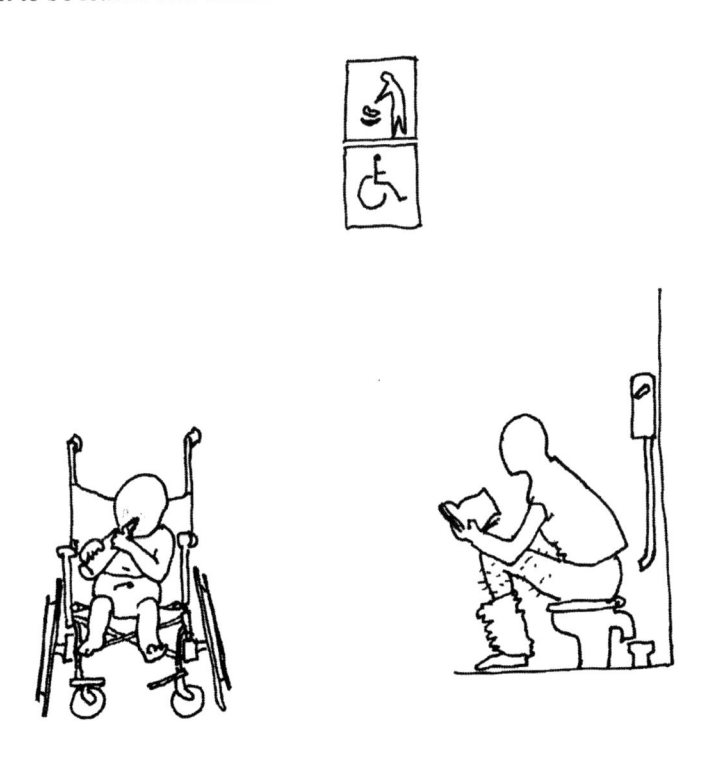

Disabled-baby toilet or disabled baby-toilet?

Public Toilets: Getting In, Getting Out, and Getting to Use Them

Getting out of Toilets

Not all toilets are so small; some are over three times the size of my bedroom. (No wonder Americans call them 'rest-rooms'. Not knowing this, I was touched by the thoughtfulness when, on my first visit to the USA, my hosts suggested I might like to use the rest-room. I expected a sofa to lie down on, but could find nothing better than the basin counter - don't other cultures have odd habits!)

Generous size doesn't automatically make toilets problem-free. They're usually easy to get into, but not necessarily easy to get *out* of. One in particular had a door that opened in. I was able to lean forward and (just) reach the handle. But how could I open the door? The wheelchair was in the way. Leaning forward, I couldn't reverse with one hand and hold the door with the other. Or could I? After all, I *had* to get out; I had a plane to catch. With much persistence, I managed a short reverse, but then the door swung too far to the right, beyond my left hand reach. The handle slid from my fingers and we (me, the wheelchair and the door) were back to square one.

Try again. This time I opened the door a crack, jammed it ajar with one crutch, reversed a few inches, pulled it a little wider and fed through the handle of the other crutch so I could hook it onto the door. I then reversed eighteen inches, set the brakes on and pulled the door to about forty-five degrees open. So far, so good, but not good enough! The wheelchair still wouldn't fit through. How could I reverse another eighteen inches and pull the door to ninety degrees? I needed two hands to reverse straight and wasn't sure my teeth were strong enough to pull the crutch. Also crutches don't taste very good - neither the aluminium nor the plastic bits. The rubber ferrule is the only tooth-friendly bit, but as I know where its been, it's the bit I would least like in my mouth.

Still needing one hand for the door-holding crutch, I tried a one-handed reverse but the wheelchair pivoted to the wall and would go no further. To free it, I had to go forward and immediately lost my precious eighteen inches. Back to square one-and-a-quarter.

Try again. This time I jammed the crutch under my armpit. Again, initial success, but once full pull had came on the crutch, both wheels skidded on the well-cleaned (or not so well-cleaned, greasy) floor. Now I was really stuck. Stuck, and still had a plane to catch. Fortunately, at this point, somebody passed in the corridor outside, noticed my predicament and rescued me.

Lesson to be learnt: If at first you don't succeed, try, try... and try to always arrange a nearby stranger.

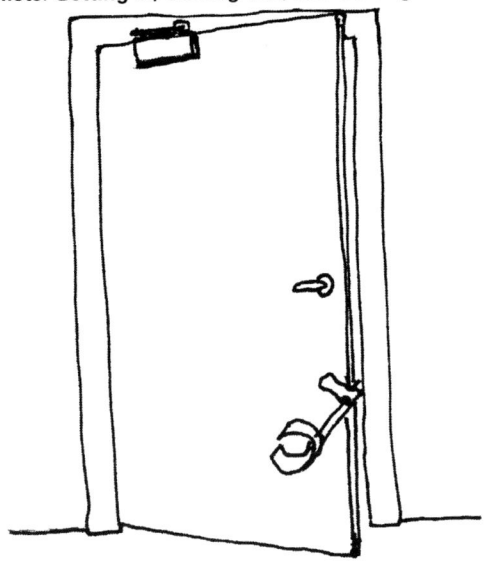

Public Toilets: Getting In, Getting Out, and Getting to Use Them

The international sign for "Let me out!"

Adventures in Toilets

Even less problematic toilets aren't always entirely problem-free. After using the toilet, it's quite nice to wash my hands. (Indeed, there's often a little notice ordering me to do so.) I therefore pull myself to the basin and turn the tap. Some basins have single taps (for one-handed people) which turn first to cold and then only to hot when fully open. (This hot-cold trick is obviously for thermal-stimulation therapy.) For water-economy and ease of washing, these are spray-taps. Spray-taps have tiny nozzle holes. Just like the thumb-on-hose trick, these jet water quite hard. This can be simply overcome by pressure adjustment, but usually isn't, so the water-jet is powerful. This is deflected by the basin lip into my face. After a thorough face and glasses wash, the surplus drains down my chest, between my legs and into the pond-shaped, waterproof wheelchair seat. Unfortunately, I move quite slowly so have been well washed by the time I can turn the tap off. Fortunately, the pressure is usually less severe and the water only reaches my lap. It now merely looks as though I didn't get to the toilet in time.

Now the soap. Only my right hand is strong enough to squeeze the dispenser and my left hand won't turn over to receive it. So I try to squeeze soap onto my right palm. This takes some contortion. As the dispenser is always mounted beside the basin, a mound of soap accumulates on the floor - dangerous if I'm on crutches, and a possible explanation for slippery floor syndrome - or, if I'm lucky, on my toe. As I can't reach this, it isn't so useful and I'm not really so lucky. Much stretching and contortion and some soap lands on (the edge of) my palm. But quick as a soapy flash, it slides down my arm to the elbow. As this is under my shirt, it's no use here - except for elbow lubrication. Nor is it even comfortable. Well, at least I can have a water-only wash - even if I must wash my crotch as well as my hands!

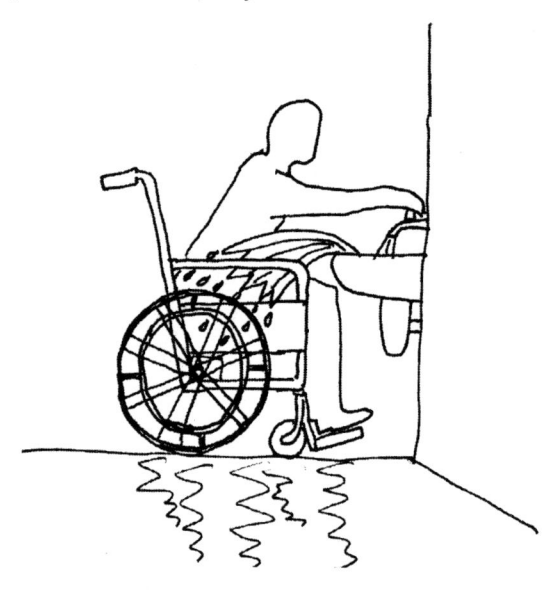

Many washbasins offer a complimentary crotch-washing service.

If I'm on wheels, I usually lean my crutches in a corner. Anywhere else and they fall on the not-convincingly-hygienic floor. But crutches like to fall - it seems to be their specialty. Hence, my contortions in trying to reach the soap can easily dislodge them. So much for hygiene! Why bother with soap? But this isn't all. If they fall behind the wheels, I'm stuck. The basin prevents forward motion; the crutches, rearward. The soap is still out of reach but my priorities have changed. Escape is now foremost in my mind. Desperate prisoners even find sewers attractive - but I hope it won't come to that. Sewers aren't made for disabled travel. So .... much maneuvering a quarter inch at a time and half an hour - and much hammering on door - later, I'm free.

Lesson to be learnt: eat sandwiches *before* going to the toilet. After all, I may never get out, and would hate to die of starvation - even though deferred gratification is meant to be good for character development.

There is also the small matter of using the toilet itself. Usually there is a fold-down handrail. Usually this is folded up. Fortunately, it's easy to get it down - all you have to do is lift it to disengage the lock, then swing it down. Easy if you're not disabled. Such handrails are steel - strongly made, so reassuringly heavy. When you're not strong or steady on your feet, however, you can only lift them by standing exactly in front. Anywhere else is off-balance. This means the heavy steel rail sledgehammer-swings down towards the one piece of my anatomy I least want it to hit.

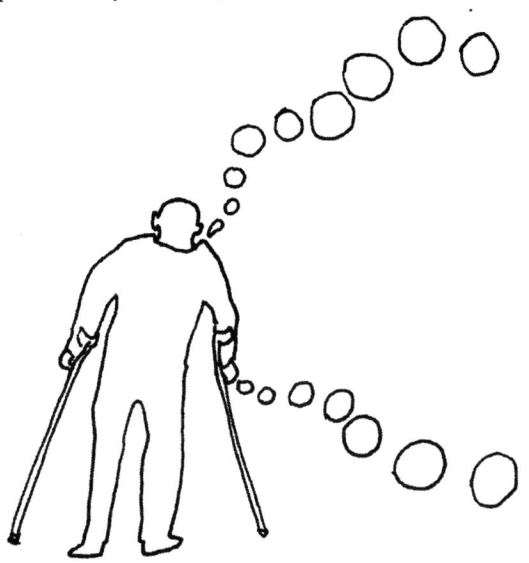

The advantages of soapy elbow.

Lesson to be learnt: toilets are high risk locations. In fact, as so many heart-attacks occur on toilets, even domestic bathrooms are dangerous!

Even the most modern toilets can have problems. Warsaw airport doesn't expect many disabled travellers. It only has one disabled toilet. At least, there is only one on the ground floor. There may be another upstairs, but as there are no lifts, this is of limited use. (Not exactly true: there *is* a lift connecting arrivals and departures – but this is only useful for people who don't know whether they're coming or going.) Warsaw is also a no smoking airport. Hence, whenever I've tried to use the toilet, it has always been occupied by a member of staff taking a smoking break.

Warsaw is to the east of the former iron-curtain. This boundary still divides Europe, but now as a toilet-paper-curtain. It is on the grey side. Everywhere in Western Europe has white toilet paper; everywhere in Eastern Europe has grey. Apart from this, and the air-quality (smoky), the toilet-room is luxurious - spacious, new, and with gleaming chromium safety rails. It even has an extra-high toilet - much easier to get up from. But how could I drain my leg bag into it? Even if I could raise my foot so high - which I can't - the bag would drain the wrong way. Backflow is not a very attractive prospect. Fortunately, there was a toilet-cleaning brush standing in a thoughtfully provided little bowl. The bowl only held a half bagfull, but this was better than nothing. Much better, as nothing would have been a disaster! But how to empty it for refilling? I couldn't reach low enough without falling out of the wheelchair - namely:

Public Toilets: Getting In, Getting Out, and Getting to Use Them

into the bowl. Fortunately, my friend was with me. On my own, I would have had to use the bin - the one provided for sanitary towels, syringes, cigarette ends and the like.

Now handwashing. There was a basin broad enough not to flood my lap and a luxury tap that worked perfectly. No crotch-washing this time! But the soap dispenser was at the limit of one-hand reach. I could, however, pile up soap-slurps on the edge of the basin, wipe these with a finger and thus transfer the soap to both hands.

Next: hand-drying. Naturally, the paper toweller was empty, but no matter - there was an electric hand-drier. I wheeled myself over, but before I came within reach, my feet hit the wall. Again, no matter, I could try sideways, wheeling along the wall. Now my feet hit the litter bin. If I pushed too hard, the top would come off and it would tip syringes - and maybe somebody else's disabled pee - onto my legs. In such circumstances, who cares about wet hands?

Unfortunately to get out of the toilet meant turning a round knob to unlock the door. Wet fingers slip on round knobs, so nothing for it but to wait. Frantic door-handle rattling, but wet hands take as long to dry as a cigarette to smoke, so this official would just have to miss his or her (unofficial) smoking break.

Lesson to be learnt: patience is a virtue - even in others.

Further lesson to be learnt: smoking causes stress - especially in no-smoking toilets.

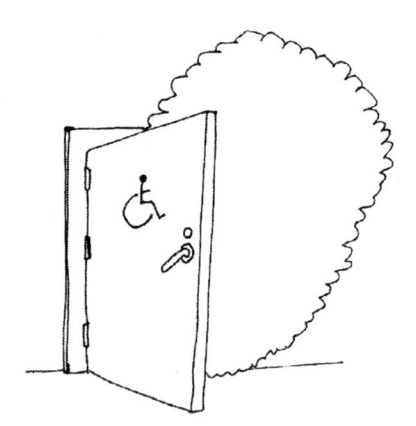

Some no-smoking airports provide toilets for staff with smoking disabilities.

Medical and other treatments

18. Hospital Life - or half-life

Conventionally, there's no treatment for my illness. There are drugs which allegedly ease some symptoms, but all drugs have side effects. Even the consultant warned me against these. How odd: when an animal is going to die, we think it best to 'put it out of its misery' by shortening its life. But when a human is going to die, we prolong life by adding misery through pharmaceutical side-effects.

There may be no treatment, but there *is* lots of investigation. I first went to my doctor when I realized I'd lost dexterity in one foot. Coupled with frequent muscle quivers and weakness in my left hand, I wondered what was going on.

I began to carefully observe my symptoms, objectively and – I hoped - dispassionately. Fortunately, school biology had prepared me for this. In the final exam, we were instructed to slit a dandelion stem and observe what happened. Five things did: watery fluid came out, my exam papers were soaked, the razor-blade was wet, the half-stems curled, and the flower looked dead. But which answer did they want? I realized I must tell the truth: "I have killed the flour." Next question: "Explain why." I wrote: "Because you told me to." I passed. If only life was so simple: skip the difficult questions, utter a few words of wisdom, and move on to better things – in that case, lunch. With these observations (about me, not the long-deceased flower) I went to my doctor. He obviously hadn't studied biology, for he couldn't swiftly decide, so sent me to the hospital consultant.

To enjoy hospitals, you have to enjoy motoring (or knitting or cooking) magazines. Also enjoy sitting in plastic chairs lined along a corridor, everyone around you looking infectiously ill. All the while, people hurry past - and over - your feet. This isn't accidental: it's Stage One of treatment. Once you can feel calm and relaxed (this takes about an hour, sometimes more) you're ready for Stage Two.

Suitably calmed by my hour's wait, I'm now summoned to a doctor. A long hobble down the corridor. It's rarely the doctor whose name was on the appointment card. This one hasn't seen me before, so like all the other doctors I've seen, he needs to examine me. Onto the couch and out come the instruments of torture: rubber hammer to hit knees, plastic spike to stroke soles of feet. Obviously, these aren't *meant* to be for torture, and usually aren't, but in the wrong hands....

At my many out-patient appointments, I had many non-diagnoses and even several diagnoses. Early on, one doctor asked me to sit down, then called

Hospital Life - or half-life

a nurse in. I intuitively realized this meant something bad. He then very gently told me that Motor Neurone Disease couldn't, as formerly thought, be ruled out. I was numb with shock. But later, I went to a neurologist who said I didn't have it. What a relief! I was just getting worse, but wasn't ill - so that was alright then! After that, doctors started guessing. Perhaps it was a neck injury. All this would need was a 'little' spine surgery to make my neck a nice shape and I would be alright - as long as I survived the neck-making-nice operation. Another doctor said: "It must have been a stroke." I asked how a stroke could have long term, slowly progressive consequences. He suggested a series of strokes. Wouldn't I have noticed them? Apparently - as I was dumb enough to ask such stupid questions - not.

This seemed as far as out-patient diagnosis could go. But there was still the high-technology method. Most importantly, **the MRI machine**.

This is big, expensive and everybody takes it very seriously. Soon I was to see why. First, you must divest yourself of anything magnetic like belt-buckles, so the machine doesn't pick you up and slam you from ceiling to floor. Then you lie on a sort of couch, your forehead strapped down. The whole assembly, me included, is now slid into a tube. Exactly above my eyes was a mirror. I could see the operator, and presumably she could see me - or anyway, my eyes. She told me not to move and not to worry. I wasn't worried; why should I be? What did they know that I didn't?

Then the noises started.

Clicks, rattles, gurgles, sounds like zap-guns in computer games, knocking, more gurgles, banging. If you believe computer-game zap-guns are the apex of technology, this may inspire confidence. I don't. So it didn't. In fact, I wondered if the machine was falling to pieces - and doing so with me inside it. As it all sounded such a bodged lash-up, it was hard not to laugh. But I had to stay still, absolutely motionless, for about forty-five minutes. It seemed, therefore, that the best thing to do would be to try to go to sleep. To aid this, I shut my eyes. "Are you all-right?" came an alarmed voice down the tube. Trying not to move my mouth, I assured her that I was only trying to go to sleep. Apparently that wasn't the normal behaviour - but what else could I do for forty-five minutes? I wasn't allowed to laugh and I certainly couldn't read in there. Well, I had read all the instructions and serial numbers on the ceiling already. They were quite boring enough to read once, and would be even more boring to re-read for most of an hour. Eventually I did get to sleep, despite the racket. I had also managed not to laugh so was allowed out. A slow slide out of the tunnel. I was unstrapped and then allowed to put my belt back on and steel back into my pockets. But now it seemed that something hadn't been done right. So... back into the tunnel for another session. This time, I knew what noises to expect; and as I had memorized the serial numbers, it was even more boring.

Hospital Life - or half-life

About a month later, I got another hospital appointment to hear the test results. Had I passed? To get to this hospital necessitated four hours driving (two each way), half-an-hour finding somewhere to park, twenty minutes finding the right part of the hospital, forty minutes waiting. All for a one-minute meeting with the consultant, in which he told me I would need to come in for a week of tests. Hospitals obviously don't know about writing letters.

Hospital appointments always seem to be at 9 a.m. on Mondays. They take about four months to happen, but the card telling me this arrives at the last minute. Usually on Saturday, so if I can't make it, I can't ring till 9 a.m. Monday. In-patient appointment cards always ask me to ring to confirm before setting out - but with the switchboard not staffed before nine and the two-hour car journey, I can't ring till I arrive at the hospital. By then, it's a bit late. Nowadays, I have a mobile phone so it's much better. I can now ring from the hospital car-park. If the appointment has been cancelled, at least I am saved the ten minutes it takes to get out of the car, twenty (for someone else) to find the department and, nowadays, forty to be wheeled to it.

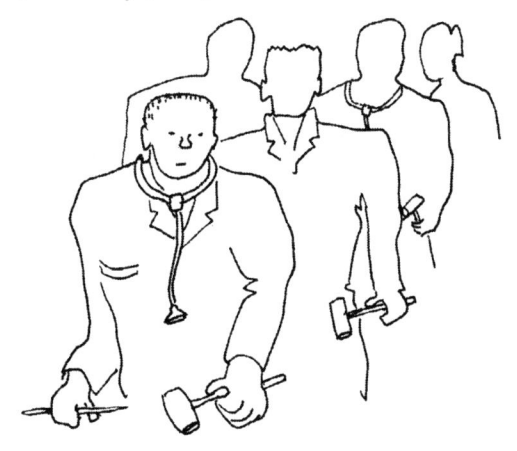

Quantum physicks: lots of doctors.

When in hospital for a week of tests, about three students would troop in to examine me each day. At last I understood what quantum physicks means: lots of doctors. As most handled me roughly, I assume patient care isn't taught in medical school. Perhaps they teach rugby in its place. Instead of tickling the soles of my feet, they would scratch them. Typically, the first one would move my stiff arm as far as it would go - but it would only go that far when forced. (Rugby is a useful skill here.) This meant that the pain in my seized shoulder would make the arm go limp. The next student would then ask me to lift my arm. As I now couldn't, he would do it for me. More pain, more limp arm - and, unfortunately, one more medical student. In the whole week, only one thought to ask how I was, what was wrong, what hurt and what she may or may not do. As it happened, she was the only one who didn't look like a rugby player.

Lesson to be learnt: rugby may be good for health (anyway for health-care professionals), but is less comfortable at the receiving end.

These tests, I began to realize, were tests for the student doctors. But there were also tests for *me*. Real - namely: machine-based - tests. These started with a chest X-ray. This was just for luck; nothing was (at that time) wrong with my chest. Then I had to give (actually, they took) eight little bottles of blood. There were also more high-tech tests. The consultant stuck alarmingly long electrode needles into my thighs, then passed current through them and looked at his TV screen to see how I responded to the electric shocks. A somewhat pointless experiment as, long before any test, I could have told him I wouldn't enjoy this. Next came an electrode wristband. This also gave me electric shocks while yet another consultant looked at *his* TV screen.

I also had an electrode glued to the top of my head. They then sat me in front of a green-gridded screen overlaying red spots. No-one thought to ask whether I might be red-green colour-blind. I am. When everyone was ready and the glue had set, someone (presumably) pressed a button, for the grid started to jump. It jumped so fast, I gave up trying to follow it with my eyes. Anyway, being colour-blind, I could no longer tell which was grid and which spots, so I'm not sure what reaction they managed to measure. Likewise, it wasn't clear if they measured my reaction to the removal of electrode-glued-to-hair. I asked if I had passed the test, but was told this information was secret, for the consultant only.

Between tests would be a day's wait in bed without any test. This presumably was to calm my nerves, but actually was a bit boring as inane quiz-shows on the super-loud television prevented reading. Moreover, I didn't feel ill enough to stay in bed. Indeed, I didn't feel ill at all - why should I? I didn't have a disease diagnosis yet.

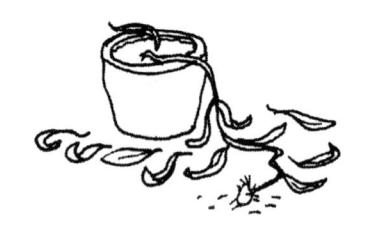

At hospital, they even asked to listen to my heart.
Unfortunately, I misheard.

I didn't learn much about my illness in hospital, but I did learn about other people's. One patient, a builder, moved even more clumsily than me and spoke with a heavy slur. The doctor asked him how much he drank. "Only twenty-three pints a day" Could that be the cause of his condition - irreversible brain-damage? "No, that isn't much. I used to drink much more." Of course without a brain any more, it's hard to link cause to effect. I also heard of someone who put thirty-five spoons of sugar in each cup of tea. I don't know which department he ended up in. Possibly cardiac, possibly mortuary, possibly sugar marketing.

In the big university hospital, to which I was next sent, there is an even bigger, especially high-status MRI Machine. As the first test hadn't shown anything wrong, I had to try again with this one. It was so powerful that the very smallest piece of metal could be dangerous. Coins could tear through pockets on one journey, and be fired through me on the reverse. Even a trouser zip could cause serious injury if I was lifted and shaken by it - indeed this is one place I would rather not be lifted and shaken by. Consequently, this meant undressing and wearing a sort of robe that looked respectable to me, viewed from the front, but is open behind - so I couldn't see how unrespectable I was. Presumably, the assumption is that as somebody's face and naked bottom aren't visible at the same time, it can't be embarrassing.

It was here, on another visit, that I got the brutal prognosis. One year to live! I wandered out in such a total state of shock that I nearly fell in the ornamental pond. Likewise I wasn't at my safest driving home. The consultant should have said: "You'll have a year to live if you survive today - good luck (with today)." In fact, I've already lived longer than a year - so what a waste of all that expensive technology!

Lesson to be learnt: technology is not infallible - especially if it's modelled on Space Invaders. It doesn't even kill you as fast as it says it will.

19. Getting cured, not-cured and fleeced: Assorted Therapies

When I say my condition is painless, this is not entirely true about life. It definitely isn't true about treatments. Some hurt the wallet, some the body. Some are stressful; some leave me exhausted (which, I'm told, is good - it means they're working).

Officially – in the government's view –my condition is incurable. (This is nothing new: they told me at school that my spelling was incurable.) They should know. I've had to spend weeks at hospitals so they could definitively tell me this. But I don't like to be told what to do by governments, so I refuse to wane as fast as they expect. One year is such an unreasonable demand - how could I finish this book in so short a time?

While conventional medicine has nothing to offer, complimentary medicine has lots. A bit like weird-food-diets, there are confusingly many alternatives, many with rigid advocates. Fortunately, these aren't all one-size-fits-all Grandma's-apple-pie type cure-alls; some are sensitive to who I am and my particular ailment. Some treatments are inexpensive; some cost an arm and a leg. Being disabled already, I can't afford to lose these.

Some of what's on offer is good, has helped me; some is useless, has made me poor. How can you tell the difference? It has been my experience that the more useless a therapy is, the more expensive it usually is. If it costs your whole life savings, it's virtually guaranteed not to work - but then, how could it? You have been proved incurable. In fact, you've proved it yourself by spending so much you can't afford any other kind of therapy. There are lots of plausible life-savings-expensive therapies around. They may well work, but I'm cautious of all-or-nothing gambles. Am I too cautious to get cured? Or is it just that I don't like to be sadistic to poor Wallet?

I've had many complimentary medical treatments and my deterioration has slowed to around a tenth of its earlier rate. With such varied therapies, often concurrent, it is hard to assess each objectively. Some seemed to make a difference, some not. Some I discontinued because I couldn't afford them, some because they were too hard to get to, some didn't seem to do anything, and some I'm still continuing with.

Electro-Neural Massage

The first person that said she could help my condition used a Skenar device (self–controlled-electro-neural-automatic-response: CKEHAP in Russian – which means the same and sounds the same, so should have taught me never to judge by appearances). This was developed for the space programme because a full range of medicines would be too heavy. (Every kilo taken into space costs a kilo of gold - hence no room on board for the thousand mini-statues of Lenin

Getting cured, not-cured and fleeced: Assorted Therapies

needed for scattering on the surface of the moon.) Moreover, sputniks, like our planet, are closed bio-systems. Without elaborate bio-processing many pharmaceuticals would re-circulate in space capsule air – just as they do on earth. We know this from the way they survive sewage treatment to turn up in drinking water. On earth, this has limited consumer appeal; in space, limited Hero-of-the-Soviet-Union appeal. While this might mean cosmonauts cured of everything before they even got ill, it would also mean cosmonauts with every kind of medical-drug side-effect known to man (or, as it was a Russian space programme, known to dog).

Unlike Western medicine with its kit-of-parts bias, Russian medicine is more energy-system based. The Skenar device measures the electrical resistance of the skin and its wavelength vibrational pattern. It recognizes aberrations in this pattern and by delivering small electric shocks, thousands of times a second, dampens these to re-establish normal healthy patterns. It looks like a TV remote controller and is similarly powered by small batteries. It is, however, more vicious. TV remote controllers don't bite. This does. It feels like being stroked with a pin, and is used on the acupuncture meridians in banded zones up the body - hence a lot of stroking. Normally I would not recommend stroking with pins, but I felt this treatment had a beneficial effect. Unfortunately the costs of travelling to London and taxis to appointments so exceeded the cost of treatment that I had to discontinue.

Kosmed is a similar device. (Kosmonaut (or kosmodog) medicine: КОСМЕД in Russian. This sounds and means something different from СКЕНАР, but *is* indistinguishable. Perhaps this should have taught me never to judge at all.) Actually it is *identical*, but when Russian scientists discovered capitalism two separate teams took out patents, signed contracts and left Western importers to fight it out in the courts. My Skenar treatment sessions were intuitive and long and carried out by a new-age dancer. The Kosmed ones were done by a doctor, short and precisely targeted. They cost about the same, were equally uncomfortable, equally effective and equally hard and expensive to get to.

I did eventually discover a practitioner nearer to home, but he required me to start 'clean' – which meant a coffee enema. Quite simple to do – according to his instructions: make coffee, put in bag provided, hang on hook, lie on floor, insert tube in rectum, open tap and as soon as the bag is empty, take up preparatory position on toilet. Personally, I think it would be less painful if the coffee cooled first. For me, however, there was one snag: I wouldn't be able to get up. Lying on the bathroom floor till rescued, didn't seem very appealing. Lying face down while the enema took effect all over that same floor was even less appealing. And anyway what a waste of good coffee!

Both Skenar and Kosmed practitioners didn't stop at pin-stroking, but also gave me homework. For one I had to repeat fifty times a day "I am healthy, wealthy and wise." Unfortunately, after spending life-savings on whiz-kid doctor (of him, more later), it was hard to convince myself that I was wealthy. Nor was I sure I had been wise to so finance his whizzing. That left Healthy in a somewhat shaky position.

For the other, I had to imagine the person to whom I felt the most (buried) anger, standing beside a cat. (It wasn't so important to also be angry at the cat.) Pointing accusingly, and with a voice whiplashing with venom, I should shout "Don't let me ever, ever, ever, catch you using *my* toothbrush to clean *that* cat's teeth, again!" This was more successful. She never did. Nonetheless, exclusive use of my toothbrush didn't quite cure me, so I extended my range of therapies.

Herbal Medicine

A friend searched the internet for ALS/MND treatments. Mostly she came up with charts I could make to measure my deterioration, ingenious cures (but no success stories) and lots of sufferers' letters. These generally ran like this: "I've fought this illness for months and I can't go on. I'm giving up. This will be my last letter." I found this rather depressing. Also, I'm not into fighting. If I didn't fight when I was agile, being crippled is hardly the best time to start to learn it. Moreover, one of the objects in fighting is to win, which means somebody will lose. There are enough losers in life - why create more? Amongst all this negative stuff, she did however find a Harley Street doctor who claimed success in treating ALS/MND with herbal medicine.

Harley Street is home to the best, or anyway the most ambitious, doctors. This one could - according to his website - cure anything. So successful – or ambitious - was he, that the illest of people came to him. And so desperate were they to be cured, that it didn't matter how disabled-inaccessible were the premises. To get in meant negotiating steps without a handrail, then opening a huge, heavy front door. Naturally, the consulting room was upstairs. Indeed, so successful was he that he hardly had time for patients - he needed to whiz on to the next one. Before treating me, he needed to know what was wrong with me. This required me to take several tests to ascertain which organs weren't performing properly. These included a sweat test, a 24-hour urine test, a faeces test and a blood test.

None of these tests were stress free. The sweat test I could take at a laboratory a mere five minutes walk away. He didn't allow for the fact that I'm slow. I didn't allow for his speediness. With two main roads to cross at my slow speed, the five minutes walk took me over twenty. Acutely aware the lab was about to close and I wouldn't be in London again, there was no shortage of nervous sweat! Next: the 24-hour urine test. Being incontinent meant that I had to carry a pee bottle around with me at all times, indoors and out. Then came the faeces test. This isn't easy and it isn't pleasant. In fact, it's one aspect of dying that definitely *isn't* fun. The pack contained a neat little fold-out cardboard tray for me to deposit a faece into. (Nurses call this a "motion" but once in the tray, I hope it won't move.) When you only have one working hand and need it to hold onto something to keep from falling off the toilet, this isn't easy. Accuracy is important. Neither half on the tray nor half on the hand is desirable. I must then empty the tray into a bottle without spilling any. Also not easy, especially while still trying not to fall off the toilet.

Blood tests may sound simple, but this blood had to be sent to a US laboratory. It must arrive by Thursday morning and be sent by 24-hour service. As 24-hour service takes 48 hours from Wales plus five hours time difference plus an hour margin for collection, this meant it must be ready for collection by 11 a.m. on Monday. The surgery could only offer me a 10 a.m. appointment so in one hour I would have to allow 5 minutes for blood extraction, 10 minutes to get into the car, 16 minutes to drive home, 10 minutes to get out of car and into house. This only allowed 19 minutes to pack the blood-samples in ice with three separate protective layers, each separately labelled - all done with one good hand and one spastic one. What if the appointment was delayed?

The stress from all these tests caused about six months deterioration in ten days. A few weeks later the results came back - about twenty pages of reports. I had no idea so many things were wrong with me. Indeed, it was a miracle that I wasn't dead - and the doctor would have worked a miracle if I still wasn't dead in six months. No wonder he was, or said he was, famous. Every single organ was functioning at least one percent below - or above - the normal (depending on what time of day the tests were performed). Of course, I knew I wasn't normal, but never knew I was *so* abnormal!

With the results in hand, it was time for another appointment with whiz-kid-doctor. A week later came two pages of faxed prescription: eighteen different sorts of herbal medicines along with telephone numbers (many incomplete) of where to get them and when and how to take them. Some had to be taken first and last thing, some with food, some half an hour before, some half an hour after, others exactly in between, meals. Nor were they easy to get. There were two mail order sources in Britain and two in America. Only one thing could be got from a local chemist, but as it had recently been added to the poison list, it now couldn't. Most things, even this poison - sounded harmless enough. But not the thigh patches from America. The company that made these wouldn't sell them without an American doctor's prescription. They did, however, fax me product details. There was a quarter-page of possible side effects including skin burns, convulsions and death. Why take quarter of a page to get to the point? Surely of all side effects, death is the most significant. Who cares about the others if you're dead? Much transatlantic telephoning, many faxes to whiz-kid-

Getting cured, not-cured and fleeced: Assorted Therapies

doctor and a few incomplete replies faxed back. I eventually found an American doctor, who, at great expense, would give me a prescription after a formality of a telephone consultation. I balked at the price. Whiz-kid-doctor, ('legal') pills and phone bills had already cost six months' income. Unfortunately, despite hearing a news-item on a one-legged bank-robber, I felt too slow to rob a bank. (Anyway, he failed; his artificial leg fell off.)

Neurotically watching the clock and popping 42 pills a day in different combinations made normal life impossible and the stress made me another six months worse. I had now deteriorated twelve months worth in one month, so if he cured me now, instead of just making me even worse, it really *would* be a miracle. The first renewal of all these pills finished my savings, so after four months with no visible improvement I didn't renew them a second time, and discontinued the course.

Two years later, I went to another herbalist practice, highly recommended by friends. This was a partnership: a diagnostician with a gadget that measured the vibrational frequency of my organs, and a herbalist. The diagnostician had immense faith in her gadget - and certainly the first course of herbal medicine appeared to have some effect. The medicine wasn't very nice. This, perhaps, was only to be expected. After all, the Victorians believed the worse a medicine tasted, the better it was for you - an attitude they applied to all aspects of life. The pills, however, were even worse. Some, I couldn't swallow, so had to chew. This was the only way, so however foul, I just had to grin (or grimace) and bear it. But these weren't just foul; they turned to gum, sticking to my tongue where they burned and burned. I didn't like these pills. Each subsequent visit found new things wrong with me. And each course of medicine had decreasing effect. There were, however, no decreases in cost, which wasn't cheap. When the diagnostician's confident claim for a 90% cure rate (and the 10% not cured were only not cured because they hadn't followed her dietary instructions) had lapsed into "maintaining my quality of life", I thought it time to save money again.

Currently, I am enjoying a third type of herbal treatment. Actually, 'enjoying' is too strong a word as this involves drinking green sludge. As a powder, this smells very like herbal supplement for cows. It probably is the same stuff, but, packaged for humans, is ten times the price. Mixed with water it makes a drink, but with a gritty paste at the bottom. The taste is palatable - anyway for cows. But the gritty sludge makes me gag. On the instructions, it suggests this is good for losing weight. "Use as a meal replacement, as often as you like." In my case, this is never. I'm not drinking it because I *like* it, but because it is meant to help, or at least, strengthen me. Sometimes, with cures like this, I wonder if it is worth being ill!

Lesson to be learnt: Getting stronger isn't always fun.

I do believe in herbal medicine - it has thousands of years experience behind it. I am, however, less convinced by whiz-kid impresarios. Traditional herbalists always found their herbs nearby. In fact, there is a view that every ailment is, at least in part, related to environment, so the remedy can also be found in your immediate surroundings. Pills made of ingredients from all over the world break this link. Also I feel pill popping never addresses more than the physical (hence superficial) side of illness. Are there charlatans out there? Undoubtedly. But the practitioners I saw definitely weren't charlatans. They believed in what they were doing. Hence their high success rates. When both doctor and patient believe in them, placebos can be 70% successful.[1] That's better than pharmaceuticals! It should be cheaper too. But, unfortunately, even if better - or no worse - it certainly wasn't cheaper in these cases! Unfortunately again, complete belief is also blinding. (When I was a child I was told 'blind faith' was good. Not a view I now share.) Hence complete belief in things is a major reason why they fail. So confident are their proponents, that they omit to rigorously self-question, so their treatment isn't always appropriate.

Lesson to be learnt: Sometimes listening is more important than knowing.

Additional lesson to be learnt: Don't be over-confident in over-confident people.

Homeopathic Medicine

Whereas herbal medicine stimulates or moderates organ processes, homeopathic medicine aims to induce the body itself to establish balance. Homeopathy works on the principle that 'like cures like'. A substance is chosen that produces symptoms typical of the ailment being treated. (But what do they make constipation remedy from?) It is then so diluted (by 'potentising' technique) that nothing of it physically remains, except its symptom-tendency. The symptoms induced stimulate therapeutic counter-balancing processes in the body. This, of course, is nonsense to conventionally-minded doctors. How can pure water cure anybody? Recent research on the molecular structure of water, however, shows it exhibits 'memory' - another ridiculously non-credible charlatan-claim, were it not that computers depend on similar infinitesimal impurities and molecular memory.

I have seen - and myself experienced - dramatic results from homeopathic medicine. But – as slowly developing conditions tend to respond slowly - not with this illness. Anything that's working is slow – like me.

Lesson to be learnt: water can be good for you. As homeopathic remedies are '100% water', they can be good too.

Getting cured, not-cured and fleeced: Assorted Therapies
Anthroposophical Medicine

Anthroposophical medicine starts with this homeopathic base, but also seeks to address underlying causes. Whatever the illness, these are specific to the individual. Unlike conventional medicine, which is interested solely in the 'illness in the person', anthroposophical medicine focuses on 'the person in the illness' - crucial to understanding why we got ill, and what to do about it. This holism leads to multi-strand therapy. At the clinic[2] to which I go annually, this includes (for me), as well as homeopathic medicines and injections, herbal baths, compresses on my organs, warm beeswax pads on the spine, eurythmy, painting, rhythmical-massage and four long sessions with a doctor.

This isn't just pampered luxury. Once you recognize that illness may itself be healing deeper ills, you can view it in a different light. This gives rise to a lot of extra-curricular laughing. In fact, nowhere have I ever laughed so much. As most of the patients have cancer and most of the remainder either continual pain or chronic depression, you might not think there's much to laugh about, but it seems there is. Indeed, the funniest person I have ever met was recovering from brain surgery. After her operation, the surgeon had said: "The good news is that you're not dead. The bad news is that the operation to remove the tumor was not successful and you have only a month to live." A year later, after two visits to this clinic, there was no trace of the tumor. Not surprisingly, I highly recommend this place.

Amongst the medicines and practices I was to continue at home were 1.0 ml homeopathic injections. When I first started these, I could do them myself. I was given an orange to practice on (poor thing - it wasn't worth eating afterwards!) and a few syringes to get started. These are calibrated 0-100, which I misread as 100 ml. When I came to buy more, no chemist stocked 100 ml syringes. Only when I was referred to a vet and saw their size – almost quarter of a pint: possibly painless for an elephant! - did I realize my mistake. This made me quite glad that I *hadn't* been able to get them.

Lesson to be learnt: Careful observation is safer than reading numbers.

By the time of my second course, I needed someone to inject me. I knew now which needles my carer should get – but these were no easier to come by! Chemist after chemist refused to serve him, until at last he came to one that gave him a free druggy pack complete with condoms and instructions of where to find safe veins for easy shooting up. The ratio of condoms to needles was low, presumably reflecting heroin induced lack of potency – or indeed interest in life.

Getting cured, not-cured and fleeced: Assorted Therapies

I was pleased with these free gifts (anyway the syringes), but in the third pack these changed from slim insulin needles to huge ones. Comparing these with draughting pencil leads, these were 0.8 mm thick – thicker than some nails for fine joinery. I assume this was an attempt to deter heroin usage. In my case, this was successful.

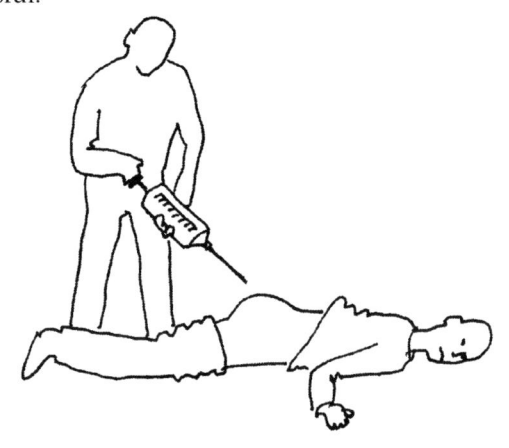

The right sized syringe hurts less.

Of the six people who have injected me to date, not all were equally dexterous. One didn't get all the air out. Only for intra-venous injections could this be fatal (why in films is the evil doctor always so careful in preparing a lethal injection?) With a sub-cutaneous injection, the main effect is a little under-skin air bubble, which delicately farts through the puncture wound. One, attempting not to hurt me, always injected at a shallow angle but, as pain nerves are near the surface, this actually hurt more. Also, it made alarming-looking - but harmless - little medicine bubbles under the skin. These couldn't fart, but could squirt. One, failing to understand my defective voice when I asked him to inject at thirty degrees, did it vertically – this is nearer to nerves and veins. Fortunately he missed both. One was so speedy he frequently dropped needles – but always caught them just before they hit the floor. Or just after, but so fast that I couldn't see it. As a former tank driver, he had a somewhat rough-and-ready approach. I didn't mind the ready bit, but wasn't so sure about the rough. I feel more at ease with more competent injectors. While, for chronic conditions, some homeopathic remedies work so slowly that you don't know if they are working at all, these injections brought warmth to my legs and feet within a week or so.

Lesson to be learnt: More haste, more screams.

Additional lesson to be learnt: Speed does not always inspire confidence.

Acupuncture

Acupuncture aims to re-open blockages to the flow of energy (chi) around the body. As acupuncture needles are very fine, they should be less painful than syringes. But not always. Some give strong 'electric–shock' sensations. Needles on the toes feel like they hit bone and are most unpleasant. Sometimes indeed, my acupuncturist asks if the needle hurts *enough*. If not, she tries again!

Needles, however, aren't the only painful aspects. To put them in my feet, the acupuncturist must take my socks off. Normally, this doesn't hurt. But unfortunately, my urine-bag is fastened around my right sock: one strap in view, one out of view. This means that when the sock is pulled off, the bag comes too. I don't mind that, but to the bag is attached a tube. This also gets pulled. To the tube is attached an important part of me. This too gets pulled. This *does* hurt - and risks bodily damage I could do without. But, despite the pain, I dare not let my body jerk lest the needles in my toes clang together and tangle. Toes may be less important than what tubes are attached to, but they too are painful! Once I am on the couch, acupuncturists have me at their mercy - so I must be good.

Lesson to be learnt: always pay bills on time.

I've been to three acupuncturists. Two didn't seem to have any effect. The other, trained in China, definitely did. My increased energy and slowed deterioration were only noticeable over a period, but other effects, like speech and digestion improvements, were dramatic. While I'm cautious about acupuncturists fast-track trained by New-Age (but Western-outlook) short courses, I definitely recommend Chinese-trained ones.

Cranial Osteopathy and Others

Some therapies appear to do nothing but nevertheless leave me exhausted. I've learnt from homeopathy that if you feel worse, that is good: the remedy is making you better. If you feel good, that too is good: it has already made you better. This means the therapist can't lose. Why don't conventional doctors do this too? Actually, they do, but they call the feeling worse mere 'side-effects'. Unfortunately, some aren't 'mere'; they don't just exhaust, but have more serious consequences and last longer - unless they kill you. By then, it's a bit late to complain.

Cranial Osteopathy works with the 'Involuntary Motion" present in all living tissue. (Nothing to do with the 'Motion' nurses ask you whether you have had.) This is subtle and complex, and includes the fluctuation of cerebrospinal fluid (which cushions and nourishes the brain and spinal chord), the movement of the skull's twenty-two bones,[3] and even intra-cellular movement. It is affected by trauma: whether injury, illness or stress. The practitioner seeks to gently re-harmonize this 'Involuntary Motion". Indeed, so gently that when my osteopath holds my ankles, small of back, sometimes head or occasionally somewhere else, she appears to be doing nothing. Nevertheless, after my first treatments I would have three days of jet-lag reaction. Jet-lag isn't really fun, but as both long and short-term beneficial effects are noticeable, it's worth it.

Microkinesilogie

Microkinesilogie is a recently developed French therapy which seeks to release trauma (both physical and psychological), locked up in the body's memory. With this, the therapist also appears to do nothing. Indeed it feels like tickle therapy as she just touches one part - initially my ankle - with one hand while the other roves fast over the body, lightly prodding. Nothing seems to happen but after forty minutes she asks me to think about and resolve biographical traumas, clearly specifying the theme and year they happened. About an hour later I (and everyone else who has done this) am overcome with exhaustion and want to do nothing else but sleep for three days. I've only been able to have four sessions, but after each my walking noticeably improved.

Energy Massage

With energy massage, another French therapy, the practitioner does even less. She doesn't even touch me, but holds her hand above my body moving it only occasionally to a new location. Result: deep sleep, followed by feeling totally limp. But next day, much more energy, more life vigour.

Lesson to be learnt: sometimes nothing is good. Sometimes doing nothing is good.

Forgiveness Therapy

In forgiveness therapy, an Estonian invention, the doctor does nothing at all. What is it about Europeans? Are they lazy - or do they know something I don't? Something about life? This was invented by a psychic doctor - the serial die-er mentioned in Chapter 1. She used to heal patients by laying on hands, but noticed most returned a year or so later with a new ailment. She realized that unless they themselves worked to heal the underlying causes of their illness, these would continue to manifest in new forms.

These causes are biographical traumas we have not released ourselves from. This we can only do through forgiveness. Easily said, less easily done. She describes the technique in her book.[4] Though simple, it is hard work. The way I work with it is this: when something or somebody upsets me, I ask myself *why* am I so upset? Viewed dispassionately, the event was small but the upset disproportionately great. What triggers to what past wounds did it touch? What did the events causing these wounds mean to me at that time? Did the people involved really mean them like that? The same action, done with different intentions, has a profoundly different effect. But we never really know someone else's intention, only what we perceive it to be. Why did they do it like that? Where, with what emotional baggage were they coming from? Once I can understand them, it is easier to accept their faults, fallibilities and mistakes. This done, it is easier to forgive them.

Why hadn't I thought of this before? From my neighbours, I had already learnt that petty irritations – however infuriating, are just.... petty. Good neighbourliness is much more important. Once I started accepting others' less-than-perfections, life became so much easier. Even dubious medical treatments, even weird food (almost) did.

Has this cured me? No. Has it healed me? Certainly it has transformed my life, adding happiness and shrinking pain. Has it slowed my deterioration? Probably. It is certainly much slower than before I started this process.

Lesson to be learnt: Healing is not the same as cure. Cure from illness may leave causes unhealed – so setting the scene for a new illness. Searching so long for a cure, blinded me to the fact that illness, itself, can heal.

Water Therapy

Amongst other therapies, I was persuaded to take a water cure. This means drinking lots of water: three litres or more a day. Clearly this is good for washing kidneys and is a delight in hot dry climates. In a cold damp one, however, there must be better ways to stem incontinence.

Bee Therapy

I never knew bees needed therapists, but a friend in the States told me about bee therapy and arranged contact with a beekeeper. I had heard of talking to bees to free yourself of all troubles – painless as long as the bees are in a good mood (no thundery weather, no smell of horses, no clashing colour combinations, no sweat or smell of fear - and don't tell them things that upset them; bees, for instance, aren't keen on adultery. They never do it). But this wasn't about talking, nor about honey or even just about having bees around – but about stinging. This also is a therapy where I do nothing - the bees do all the work. Hence only worker bees will do. Being workers, they are, of course, female.

This involved twenty stings a session. (In the States, some bee-fanatics take fifty stings each day. Some of these b... fanatics are even still alive.) For me, however, there are 'only' three sessions a week: Mondays, Wednesdays and Fridays. (Bees need weekends off.) Apparently after two years I can expect to see my deterioration slowing down. Certainly so many stings provide a good incentive not to need a third year. The bees, held in hairgrip tweezers, are placed on either side of the spine and exhorted to sting me. Most are willing but a few

Getting cured, not-cured and fleeced: Assorted Therapies

are too nice, gentle or pacifist to do so. No mercy for conscientious objectors; they're pressed until they have no choice!

The beekeeper trained my friend and she trained my daughter. Each was terrified (not surprisingly!) of bees and, as stinging means death to a bee, hated the thought of killing them. But each overcame her fear, so this therapy is obviously good for them. Whether it's good for me I can only answer in two years.

The technique starts with catching bees – putting a special box over the flight hole at dusk and tapping the hive to annoy its occupants. Too early, too loud a tap or bees in bad mood (e.g. Friday night after pub) means too many angry bees. This keeps my daughter fit. She is now a quality sprinter. Next the bees are quietened down by twenty minutes in the fridge. Forty-five minutes of television soap opera later, they're nearly dead of hypothermia and hardly notice being tweezered. One hour later (a better TV programme) they *are* all but dead.

Hypothermia symptoms include grumpiness - namely stinging - and atypical behaviour - namely not stinging. Mostly, however, they're clasped in each others' legs, fast asleep. Nevertheless, a few escape and cannon around inside the lampshade till exhausted, when they drop out on, or near, her or me. More terror. Or next morning a lonely bee on the floor finds my foot and crawls up inside my trousers. Wondering if you will be stung is much more frightening than knowing that you will be!

Freezing bees to death is cruel. Moreover they need to be awake to sting - which kills them. Poor frozen bees. Poor stinging - hence self-sacrificing - bees. Why couldn't they have been left in peace so they could work themselves to death in three weeks like any normal bee? Life just isn't fair!

Lesson to be learnt: like pearls and honey, beestings - and most good things in life - are bought at the price of sacrifice and often pain.

Then the stinging. Does it hurt? It's nice to be told how brave I am, but as there are (fortunately) fewer pain nerves in the back, mostly it doesn't. A few stings do the red-hot poker thing, but most are just bramble pricks. (I've already been here before with electro-pin therapy: Skenar and Kosmed.) Normally I try to think about something else, but when my stinger asks: "has it stung you yet?" I have to concentrate on the burning area on my back and distinguish sharp bee toenails from hard, cold tweezers. Then, when the bee finally does sting, I certainly feel the jab. Consequently, the worst pain is caused by the pacifist bees.

Lesson to be learnt (again): life isn't fair.

Bee-sting therapy should continue as an uninterrupted course. Two whole years of unrelieved stinging. This means travelling abroad presents problems; apparently bees aren't welcome on planes least they escape. (It seems that security officials are worried about terrorists with bee weapons). Nor would it be kind to the bees to pass them through the X-ray machine. So why not use foreign bees? Unfortunately, these hibernate in winter. (Are they, like foreign (do-nothing) therapists, lazy? Or sensible?) This means no bees abroad in winter, so the vital course continuity is broken. All is not lost however; the beekeeper made me a mixture of beestings and honey. Why couldn't he have done this before? All those months of needless pain! But when the mixture arrived, I was less sure! The pot was marked:

DANGER
Bee-venom–honey
Never exceed half a level teaspoon

I was told to keep it upright at all times during travel. As other people take and park my hand luggage and fail to understand me, this is impossible to control; just a stress to add to the many others when travelling. Fortunately, the honey was semi-thick - in other words, only semi-runney. (It couldn't be too thick as thick honey is, of course, made by thick bees. Runny honey, on the other hand, is the product of bees that have the runs.)

Before taking, venom-honey must be deep stirred, to ensure I eat both venom and honey. Pure honey would make me no better, so I would die. Pure venom would kill me. After stirring, I must now estimate half a teaspoon from the semi-runny honey all the way up the spoon handle. Too little is ineffective, too much and it will kill me - again! This however would eliminate all symptoms, so proving it works. Nonetheless, this would not be the cure of my choice. Come back beestings!

Does this work? Ask me in two years time. After 6,240 stings, I will either know or be fed up with being stung. In the meantime, I can at least post a warning to burglars on my gate: "Beware of the bee."

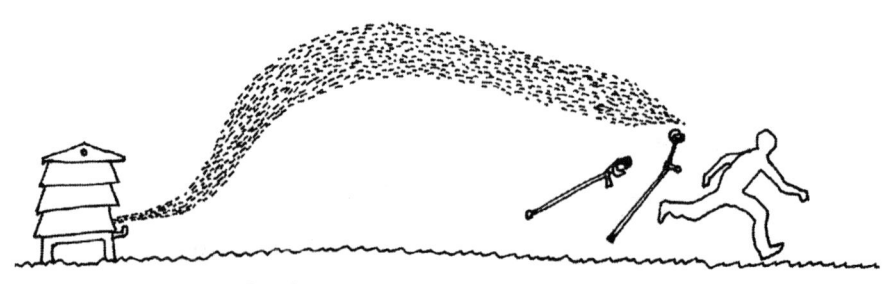

Bee therapy can achieve dramatic results.

Getting cured, not-cured and fleeced: Assorted Therapies

Kriotherapy

This I met as a Polish invention, but actually it's Japanese – via German. (This should have given me confidence, but as I still can't understand my Japanese clock/calculator instructions, I wonder what might have been lost in translation.) Like American apple-pie (in this case: Polish vodka), it allegedly cures everything. It's especially good for nerves: even the most excitable people go quiet when frozen solid.

All you have to do is don protective clothing, including something to breathe through, and get frozen to minus two hundred and sixty degrees Celsius for three minutes. Unfortunately, when I get cold, everything seizes up so I'm too stiff to look at my watch, let alone move a foot – which anyway is encased in iced urine (the plastic bag wouldn't survive -250°). Hence, once in the cold chamber, I would be there for good. Insofar as I would never experience any symptoms again, it certainly would cure me. Also, I would be pre-chilled in preparation for the fiery furnaces. This however, would be yet another of my non-favourite ways to go. Nonetheless, I had been prescribed this therapy. Unfortunately, the same day, I read that some doctors support euthanasia. This did not boost my confidence.

Such were my fears. In the event, however, I was 'only' frozen to -120° C – half way to absolute zero, where even atoms are too cold to move. Some people think this is a crazy idea, but in engineering terms it makes good sense: the heat removed (for which patients pay) heats the swimming-pool (for which swimmers pay). This makes it an eco-friendly (but not patient-friendly) therapy.

Despite dreams of the freezer doors freezing shut, the most dangerous bit was *getting* there. The Kriotherapy Department was in the rehabilitation wing of a sports centre. The only disabled accessible route took a 150 metre detour with five steep ramps. (These alternated up and down in quick succession, some at 1:2 gradients). It also crossed the shot-put and javelin range. Fortunately, most sportsmen throw shot, hammers and javelins accurately. Only a few miss. Fortunately again, most people can twist to avoid the miss-aimed ones. Unfortunately, I can't. Hence my nerves were always in need of freezing calm.

When wearing only shorts, socks, gloves, ear-band and face-mask, -120° C is unimaginably cold. Indeed, I would not recommend anyone to even *try* to imagine it. I was prescribed ten sessions. The doctor assured me that *everyone* felt better afterwards. He was right. No more -120°! I felt wonderful! Who wouldn't?

Did it work? Only after the course, did he tell me I must wait and see. But if it didn't work, he recommended more sessions. Such are the advantages of privatised medicine: if something doesn't work, buy more.

Lesson to be learnt: cool is not *always* good.

Getting cured, not-cured and fleeced: Assorted Therapies

Over-therapy

Almost every day I discover more therapies out there. Some – like Aurovedic medicine – have multi-millennial pedigrees. Some – like hyppotherapy – sound intriguing. (Less intriguing when I discovered this involves riding horses, not hippos.) Some are distinctly promising, some even free. Others, like being massaged by six Florida doctors while floating weightless in warm water, are clearly expensive. The course lasts one week, but what happens when my life-savings run out? This would happen during the first session (actually: flotation). What then? Would they, without being paid for it, help me out of the tank? Drain the water for another (more financially viable) patient? Or just let me sink?

Good or bad, cheap or expensive, any more therapies mean I have no time left to *live*. I may extend my life in years, but get no minutes life out of it. Anyway, by now I'm all theraped-out. There is, however, one possibility - and I'm working on it: a development of do-nothing therapy - air-therapy.

Air-therapy

I've learnt a lot about curing and not curing. So I'm now working on a new invention: air-cure therapy. For a mere £ 10,000, this will double your lifespan. If it doesn't, I can personally guarantee a full refund. All refund applications to be applied for in person.

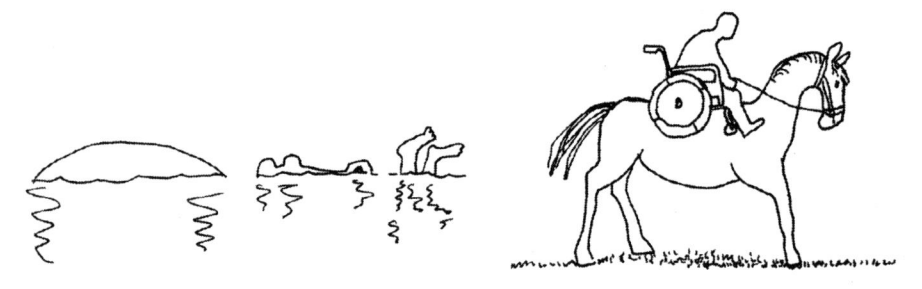

Hyppotherapy: For longevity, it's important to chose the right version.

(Endnotes)

1. Helmut Kiene: *Questioning the Dogma of the Placebo Effect*; Newsletter, the Anthroposophical Society, London, Summer 1997, and: Ian Wickramsekera *Secret kept from the Mind but not the Body*; Advances, Volume 15 No 1 Winter 1999, Fetzer Institute, Kalamazoo, Michigan, USA.
2. Park Attwood Clinic, Trimpley, Bewdley, Worcestershire, DY12 1RE, England. Tel: 01299 861444. www.parkattwood.org
3. Or twenty-nine, if you count the inner ear and throat bones.
4. Luule Viilma (1997): *A Teaching of Survival*; Luule Viilma, Haapsalu, Estonia.

Officialdom

20. Dealing with the Government

When I went to the Doctor with my broken nose, he asked if I was getting any disability benefits. I did know such benefits existed, but the only person I knew who got them was perfectly fit but prone to alcoholic bouts. Not being alcoholic, I assumed therefore that these didn't apply to me. I was assured they did. The government, it seems, wants to help – as long as it can put me in the right box. Unfortunately, being disabled is incapacitating enough. Being disabled in a box is worse.

Mindful of box limitations, I duly applied – and waited. I rashly expected something to happen, but had forgotten I was dealing with The Government.

Naturally nothing happened for three weeks. Then I received a letter in ultra-simple English (no words longer than two syllables). This letter met the 'crystal standard' for clear English. Whatever it gained in clarity, it made up for in lack of content. It took two pages to say my application would be looked at soon. Three weeks later, another identical letter and every three weeks thereafter, another. One day, however, there was a different letter: a doctor would come to examine me to ascertain whether I really was disabled.

I dreaded this test - surely like all exams there was a high chance of failure. He duly came and examined me thoroughly - as thoroughly as the six doctors and eighteen medical students before him. He then asked what I could and couldn't do. To every question I could, after some thought, work out a way of doing it. Could I make myself a meal? I had already stopped cooking, but in extremis I could put an egg in one pocket, butter in another, bread inside my shirt. This way I could take bread and butter to the table and drop the egg in the electric kettle. True, butter doesn't travel well in pockets in summer so this would be seasonal fare. I would at least be able to eat in winter. "You're shooting yourself in the foot." he told me, and wrote down that I couldn't cook. More months of waiting and then a letter telling me that I had passed: I was disabled.

Lesson to be learnt: don't worry too much about exams. As in life, worrying does nothing to affect the outcome.

As time went on I became more disabled. On one train journey the guard asked me why I didn't have a disabled rail-card. Many people more able than me did. To be eligible however I would need the next level of benefit. I applied.

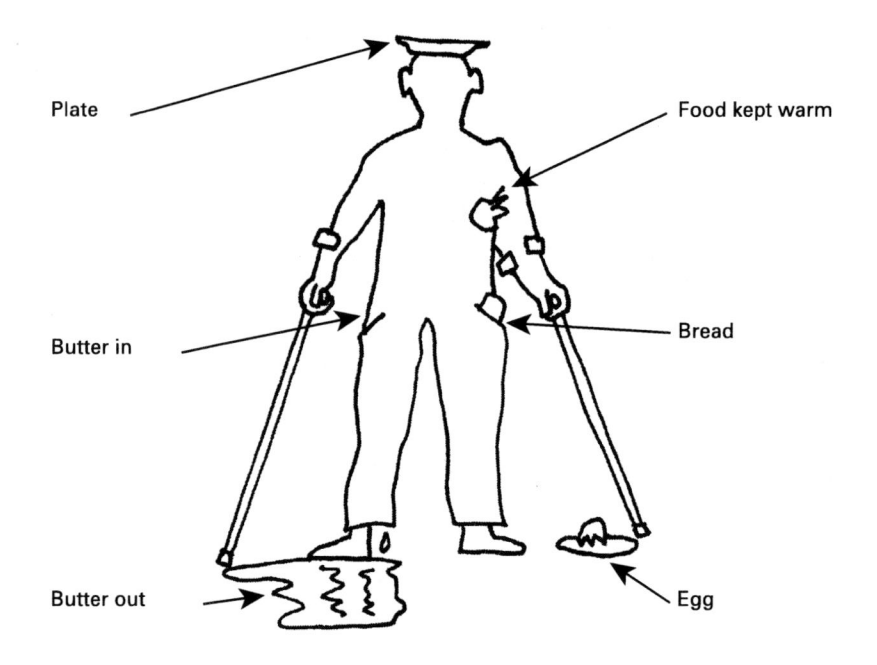

How to carry food.

More forms to get, then fill in, more letters saying nothing. Months more waiting. Then a different letter: rejection! If I disagreed with the decision, I could contest it. I did. More forms to fill in, more letters, more waiting then: another rejection.

I rang up the office, why had they rejected my application? They had caught me out with the trick question: "How long does it take to walk fifty metres?" I had answered fifteen minutes. But as I *could* walk fifty metres - even if it took a day - I couldn't be disabled. I could however appeal in court. I would. Next came a letter warning that if I proceeded I would be re-evaluated and could risk losing all benefit! This sounded awfully like a threat. So much so, that I silently vowed not to vote for the government. If they wouldn't be nice to me, I wouldn't be nice to them. Later, I discovered that governments don't even notice.

Lesson to be learnt: don't worry about governments; they don't worry about you.

The court date was fixed, only six months to wait. I realized it would be quicker to re-apply - especially as I was now six months worse than when the whole process started, which must surely strengthen my case. But no - I couldn't make another application with a court hearing pending.

Dealing with the Government

At this point my daughter wrote to our Member of Parliament. Three days later I received another letter from the Benefits Agency. 'In the circumstances' they had decided not to proceed with their court case against me (I hadn't realized they were prosecuting me for not being disabled enough - or was it for being *too* disabled?) and my application could now be approved.

Two weeks later, nine months benefit was paid into my bank account. The same week I had transferred the last of my savings into my current account to pay my son's college fees. The bank computer noticed this. On the evidence of one month's transactions I was now a big earner and big spender. The bank manager came to see me. She could offer me an account with special benefits, low interest overdraft and a book full of vouchers for half-price meals at plush, but flavourless, restaurant chains nowhere near where I live.

Lesson to be learnt: It's really true: black clouds *do* have silver (in this case paper-money) linings.

How nicely banks treat you when you are (or are thought to be) rich. How different from when you are down. When a few years earlier I had crossed my overdraft limit by twenty pounds (due to the bank's error) my whole world had collapsed. Suddenly bills I had paid, but the cheques not yet paid in, became unpaid – each adding a fifteen-pound fee to my overdraft. No phone, so no work. No professional indemnity insurance, so I wouldn't be allowed to work, even if I had any. No car insurance, so I couldn't drive; no credit card settlement, so 28% interest; and bank charges at twenty pounds a day plus interest. Within one month I would owe a thousand pounds if I spent nothing. This is more frightening than being ill, a faster road to death (by starvation) and much, much less funny. But now, thanks to the government, it was the other way round. Now I was seeing the bank's other face.

Lesson to be learnt: even heartless grant agencies are better to deal with than capitalist computers.

Other lesson to be learnt: everything works out all right in the end.

Third lesson to be learnt: the blackest situations bring the most unexpected benefits. In my case, the bank as (albeit fair-weather) 'friend'.

Fourth, and final (unless I live longer) lesson to be learnt: whether bank or government, capitalism or socialism, so long as they made life stressful, I didn't feel very forgiving. Actually, so long as I couldn't forgive, everything was stressful. But now I have forgiven them, all stress has disappeared.

Travelling

21. Trains, planes, boats and me

Flying

Airports are humour-free zones. You can be jailed for joking with security staff. This makes airports less fun. And even worse: they now insist you have your eyeball stamped into your passport. Painful! But at least they are, anyway in theory, disabled-friendly. Disabled assistance, however, is patchy. Walking off the plane in the States - in those days barely limping - I would be seized by someone with a wheelchair at the ready, even though I hadn't arranged any help. I would then be run through the airport, bag collected, ushered through immigration control, everything at high speed and ultra-efficient and courteous. I was very impressed. My pusher even politely hung around at the end to see if I needed any more help and wish me to "have a good day". Only later did I discover that for this unsolicited help he expected a $20 (now probably $50) tip.

In Europe, you don't expect to pay to be disabled. Dublin excepted. There, you have to pay for a wheelchair, but this you don't find out till it arrives at the last minute. No time, now, to walk, so if you don't have cash (they won't take a card) this could be a problem. It was.

Lesson to be learnt: life is cheaper if you don't even look the tiniest bit disabled. It doesn't pay to be ill.

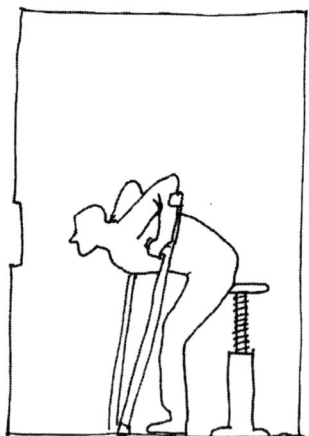

Disabled travel requires photo-identification.
Disabled-inaccessible photo-booths require ingenuity – both to get in, and for height adjustment.

When I was only walking with one stick, I discovered at Gatwick airport, London, that I could ride on a special cart, innocently peep, peeping it's way as it relentlessly mowed through crowds. Five years later, now in a wheelchair, when I asked for assistance at Heathrow (London's other main airport), I was just curtly ordered to "go over there." No-one to take me to the toilet - but then, there is a natural limit to sympathy. It would obviously be unreasonable (and uneconomic!) to ask for help onto the plane AND to be taken to have a pee. I would have to choose. Which is the more important? the more urgent? Like life, the more urgent and the more important are rarely the same!

Stanstead, London's third airport, is both better and worse. Better, because it's disabled-friendly. Worse, because trains from there to London end up in an underground station with only stairs to the surface. A journey part disabled-accessible, part disabled-thinking.

Edinburgh airport is easier to get to - initially. The airport bus can kneel close to the ground so I don't have to step high to get on. Wonderful! But when it arrives at the airport, it doesn't stop near the departures door, but in a bus-park several hundred yards away. By the time I have gotten off the bus, all the other passengers have gone. I'm left in the middle of nowhere, alone. Fortunately, there is a button I can press to ask for help. Unfortunately, it's not so easy. Can I wheel myself to it? Do I dare leave my bag while I do? (I am mindful of all the warnings that the army will suddenly appear from nowhere and detonate my previously unexploded bag.) Can I reach the button? Is my voice loud enough to reach the microphone, set for a standing person? Could my slurred speech be understood? No, No, No, No and No. Had I not a friend to help me, I would still be there. Are bus-stops my favourite place to sleep? No. And do I enjoy sleeping hunched in a wheelchair? No.

Lesson to be learnt: If you need disabled help, don't be too disabled.

It's not much fun to be forgotten either. In one airport (which should - or perhaps should not - be nameless), I was delivered by a friend, put in a wheelchair and she was told to push me to the departure lounge. But, not travelling, she wasn't allowed through security, so getting as far as the lounge was impossible. The security official told her where to park me - with assurances that I wouldn't be forgotten. I was. Various boarding calls. As airport wheelchairs are specially designed so that you can't wheel yourself, and no official was in sight, there was nothing I could do. This was not good for calmness-level. Eventually I managed to attract staff attention and was again reassured I wouldn't be forgotten. Last calls. I began to feel less reassured. Urgent calls for passenger Day. I now felt less reassured than ever. At this point, as I subsequently discovered, they took my luggage - with essential disability aids - off the plane. Finally, the check-in desk clerk arrived, very annoyed I wasn't in the departure lounge, and rushed me to the plane. Absolutely last minute, and though I had got up at 4 a.m., this was the only connecting flight that day. Had I missed it, it would have been 4 a.m. the next morning and the same risk of being forgotten all over again.

Trains, planes, boats and me

At other airports, I've waited a long, long, time and suddenly someone has arrived, breathless and flustered, to rush me onto the plane. But no-one has ever *admitted* they forgot me. Airports don't make that sort of mistake. Indeed, like banks, airports *never* make mistakes - it is always the customer's fault.

Being forgotten by taxis is a fact of life, but I also had one that refused to take my wheelchair. I protested that, folded, it's no bigger than a large case, but he was adamant - it was too large; his wife was in the car. (He didn't say how large she was.) This also was after getting up at 4.30 a.m. for a flight cancelled the previous day so now re-arranged for minimum check-in time.

There have been other problems flying. Because airports are so large, I'm invariably put into a wheelchair - whether I want it or not. In one (again, undeservedly nameless) airport, even though in their wheelchair, there were complications. After a long wait, I was speed-wheeled - once again at the last (almost forgotten?) minute - onto the bus to the plane. With weak legs after sitting immobile for two hours, I had to step onto the bus, then sit back in the wheelchair on the bus, get out of it again to step off the bus, then back into it to be wheeled twenty metres to the foot of the boarding steps. There, the stewardess said to my pusher: "He can't go on the plane." "Why not?" " We're not allowed to take anyone who can't walk up the stairs." This was not what I wanted to hear. Also, how did they think I could get home? If they didn't think I was up to walking through the airport, how could I walk six hundred miles?

All this conversation was going on a few yards away from various jet tuning-up orchestras. In my weak voice I tried to get heard. Eventually they noticed me. I suggested that I at least *try* to walk up the steps. After all, narrow steps have two handrails, so are safe(ish) if slow. (True: there is a gap in the handrails at the top, but this means there's only one place - albeit the worst one - to fall off them.) They weren't keen. What if I fell, killed myself, then sued them? I tried to explain that if I fell, it would be *I* who did it. I considered adding that if I did kill myself, I might enjoy death so much I wouldn't feel like suing - or, if I couldn't work out how to do that, haunting - them. I wasn't sure whether this would help, however. Eventually, and somewhat grudgingly, they let me try. So I didn't have to spend the rest of my life in that particular airport!

Sometimes, I'm allowed to walk down plane steps, sometimes I'm taken on a lift-wagon (usually there is a short - but alarmingly unguarded - bridge from plane to wagon, that I have to walk, all weak-legged from sitting long in a wheelchair!) Once, I was carried out by firemen. Sometimes I'm strapped into a mini-wheelchair, then carried down the steps. These have to be mini to pass down the narrow aisle. That means they are alright for mini-bottoms, but bash elbows on every armrest. On one occasion, the buckle didn't work so the straps were sort-of tied around me - 'sort-of' because they weren't long enough to properly tie. Two men, one large, one small, then lifted me and carried me down the stairs. This didn't go smoothly. The large one above pushed hard; the small one below stumbled backwards down the steps. I now regretted not walking; I would have felt much safer.

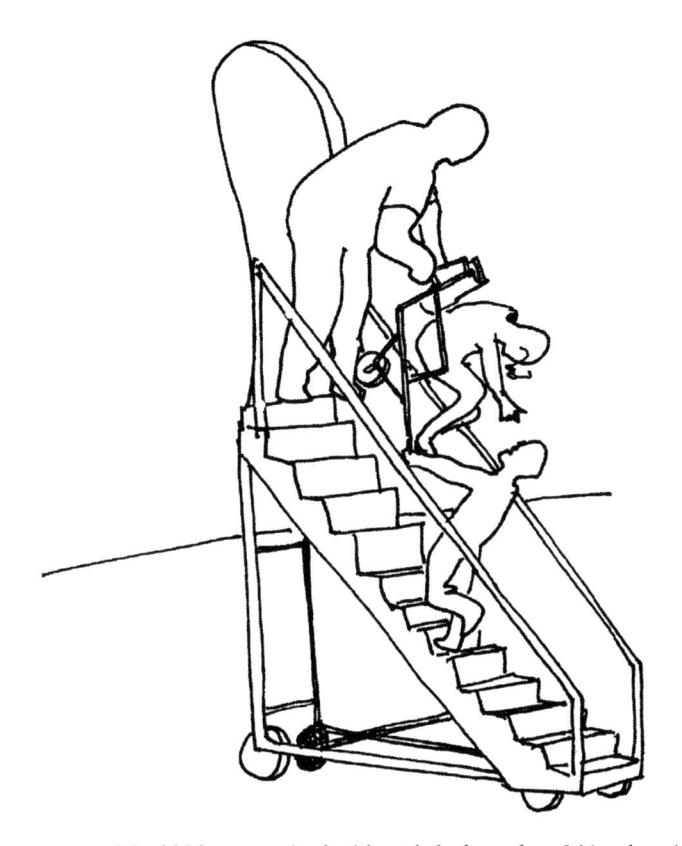

Would I have survived without help from above? Yes please!

There are also more sophisticated mini-wheelchairs, so designed that two people can 'easily' lift me from chair to seat, or the reverse. 'Easily', however, is open to human error - and 'reverse' can also cause problems. At the end of one flight, one such chair and two carriers came rushing down the plane aisle. No doubt they hoped their enthusiasm would compensate for the half-hour it had taken to find the chair. (The trouble with mini-things is that they can easily get lost.) So enthusiastic were they, that they didn't think to turn the chair to face forward like the seats. No matter - they were strong; they could turn me. One man leant over the seat back and clasped me under the armpits. The other reached in and picked up my legs. So far, so good: I was off the seat. But how to turn me? In front was seat; behind, seat-back; above, lockers. But why should they be deterred? Like me, these men clearly believed the 'impossible' is always possible. Unlike me, they also believed that force is the best method. I don't. Nor did the jammed bits of my body that were being forced. Eventually it became clear that the only way to get me into the chair would be to reverse all the way up the long aisle, off the plane, turn it, and come back backwards, possibly not at a run.

Lesson to be learnt: Even when using brute strength, 'more haste, less speed' still applies.

Further lesson to be learnt: Never tackle the impossible head-on. It's always easier if you approach it from the right direction. Indeed, it then becomes not only easy, but *possible*.

Now that I am more disabled, I get the parcel treatment. The trouble with parcels is that they don't pee. They just get parked somewhere, then rushed to another parcel park. This means that when I'm a parcel, it's hard to get taken to the toilet. As it's hard to speak, especially over my shoulder, I often have to resort to gestures and pointing. The last time I tried, however, my pusher didn't hurry me to the toilet, but stopped - not what I wanted! "Are you in pain?" he asked. "Do you need a doctor?" No, I needed a pee - but he still didn't understand. I wondered whether I should draw a picture - or whether that might contravene obscenity legislation. Are you allowed to draw anatomical pictures in airports? Or only on toilet walls?

To overcome such problems, I now carry prepared notes to show my pusher. These are requests like:

'Can you take me to the **toilet** please?'

'Can you get me a drink of **water** please?'

'Can you find someone from **disabled assistance** to help me please?'

By folding the paper line by line, I can show the message of my choice. Unfortunately people aren't used to such an unequivocal method of communication, so they usually take the paper from me, unfold it and themselves choose which message to read. Consequently, I may be brought water instead of being taken to the toilet. This is nice, but no help in an emergency. In fact, it's counter-productive.

On a recent flight, the stewards rapidly concluded that "he doesn't speak any English" - as they told each other while handing me over. (So convinced were they that when passing me to the ground-staff on arrival in Warsaw airport, these naturally assumed that I spoke Polish!) They were, however, all surprised by how quickly I could understand their loud-voiced instructions. It wasn't really necessary to repeat them four times, but just to be sure, they did. After all, I dribble, make inarticulate noises, so it's obvious I'm half-, or perhaps, quarter-witted. (This is fine. It gets me out of conversation. As I can't speak, 'conversation' is anyway a monologue.) As I obviously wasn't speaking English, it was clear I was either an imbecile or a foreigner. Consequently, they didn't need to attend to my requests, like having my briefcase in reach for the flight. After all, it was obvious I was too ga-ga to work. Without the water in my briefcase I couldn't talk at all, so couldn't argue my defence - hence they were proved right. Nor could I reach the call button, high above my seat. As I was too disabled to ask them, it didn't occur to them I might have needed help with lunch.

I didn't need help *eating* - as one of life's pleasures, I like to do that myself. But I did need help to get *at* the food. Being unfamiliar with convenience foods, I have always found plastic pillows hard to open. In the past, I used to split them with a penknife, but a penknife would transform me from a harmless, half-witted cripple to a dangerous terrorist - perhaps a member of the Cripples' Liberation Army. (But, at least I would be a terrorist who could open his lunch!) Despite crutches and a wheelchair easy to fill with explosive, I'm never allowed even a small knife - despite being too disabled to sharpen it. Fortunately, with the food comes a packet of plastic cutlery. Instead of a knife, I could use a fork. As its prongs had a napkin folded over them, some juggling was necessary before they were positioned for break-out from its bag. Once it was out, I could stab the fully inflated food-pillows. This, however, was not as easy as it may sound, for plastic forks are always blunt (terrorists aren't allowed sharp forks), while the pillow was bouncy, slippery and strong. I needed to be careful that the fork didn't slip off and stab my thigh, plumbing pipe or more sensitive anatomy. Eventually: I had success and could enjoy ('enjoy'?) the meal - now unappetizingly cold.

Next came tea. I like milk in my tea. Naturally, there wasn't any, only UHT. As this was the same colour - but not flavour - it would have to do. Opening the little UHT pot with stiff, weak fingers proved impossible. Fork (now curried) to the rescue again. I tried to jab holes in the lid. Like all food pillows, this pot was inflated into a sphere, tough and slippery, so, to keep it from springing across the plane and hitting someone in the eye, I needed to grip it hard. Fine - until I eventually succeeded in fatally stabbing it. Suddenly it became a weak, flabby, empty thing and its former contents were all over my neighbour. Fortunately, it was only UHT, not milk, so wasn't much of a waste. But my neighbour wasn't pleased. The stewardess was very solicitous to her, but with hard unsympathetic glances at the cause of all this trouble - me.

Lesson to be learnt: disabled, non-English speaking packages aren't always popular.

Normally, cabin staff are helpful and only rarely condescending. Frequently, they kindly arrange a more convenient seat for me. More convenient for them because it's less far to carry me; more convenient for my neighbours because they can get to the toilet instead of bursting beside me. This, however, means a seat change for someone not yet on the plane. Invariably, when they arrive, they aren't pleased. They show their boarding card and demand to see mine. In my slurred voice, I try to explain. All they understand is that I am drunk and refuse to move. This does nothing to improve their friendliness. Despite the wisdom in being polite to drunks - who can be as unpredictably violent as bulls - their politeness deteriorates. This minor inconvenience for them rapidly escalates into a big stress for me. But all it's about is preferring a window seat (with a view solely of wing and engine) to freedom to get to the toilet. Some people have crossed (legs) priorities.

Lesson to be learnt: In life, as in crime, what isn't big to the do-er, has much greater impact on the done-to. I need to learn that they only meant a *small* hurt, despite me feeling a big one. This also works with nicer things, like unexpected gifts. *Doing* magnifies intention many-fold.

Package-class doesn't guarantee stress-free travel. Indeed, package treatment doesn't always make things go smoothly, even for the package handlers. On one flight, I was speed-wheeled from gate to plane, crutches in one hand, boarding-card in the other. To board, however, I had to walk the last three metres. My pusher offered me his hands, but mine were full. I, therefore, offered him my crutches and boarding-card. He took the crutches and held them in front of me - not much help to get up from the wheelchair. I now had one free hand but needed two. What to do with the boarding-card? I offered it once more. Again he declined, so I put it in my mouth. This gave me two free hands, but meant I now couldn't speak at all, only gesture. Usefully (or uselessly) holding my crutches, he was no longer offering a helping arm, so I had to try to lever myself out of the wheelchair on my own. Half-way up, I felt myself pulled back. Hardly the time for a joke - and anyway, not one I thought funny! Try again. This time I got three-quarter-way up, but the wheelchair came too. At security, I had had to surrender my waist-pouch to the X-ray machine. Evidently my pusher had re-secured it to both me *and* the wheelchair. True: this is doubly secure. Unfortunately, when disabled, it's hard to walk with a wheelchair lashed to your bottom.

My mouth being full of boarding-card, I could only point. Pusher understood enough to undo the pouch buckle, but not enough to do it up again. Consequently, when I stood up, the pouch, full of valuables, fell off - fortunately not through the gap between ramp and plane. I pointed. To rescue it, he gave the crutches to someone else. (Obviously, as I was in a wheelchair, I wouldn't need crutches. Already, I had begun to wonder about his brain-power - if any.) Crutchless, I now had to hold his arm. To help me walk, he took a step back. This, of course, pulled me off balance. Pivoting from his arm, I grabbed at the aeroplane door edge - and missed, pulling *him* off balance. He called for help - the panic tone in his voice not helping my confidence - and with a steward, dragged me onto the plane. In the narrow aisle there was no space for five feet (four of theirs, one of mine) so my raised foot had the impossible task of finding somewhere to land. It failed. This meant I was totally dragged at a forty-five degree angle and pushed into the nearest seat. I wanted to tell them that I could walk if I had my crutches, but with a boarding-card in my mouth, couldn't. Anyway, I didn't have the crutches. But nor did I have my waist-pouch with money, passport and tickets.

Trains, planes, boats and me

Nor my briefcase, with the manuscript for this book. I wasn't sure which would be the greatest loss, which to worry about most. Fortunately, I *did* have a boarding-card. Unfortunately this was now half-digested.

While all this was going on, comments like "He needs medical attention when we land" and "Radio ahead for a doctor" were passing over my head. Not good for morale; and not possible to answer with a mouth full of boarding-card. But as I learnt from films, every story has a happy ending. (I also learnt how to pack: throw everything into case and shout, "I'm going". If the case won't shut, a sob is meant to help - though personally I've never found this effective.) The 'nearest seat' that I had been parked in turned out to be First-Class, so I now enjoyed an instant up-grade. This included real cutlery and glasses. (Terrorists obviously don't travel First-Class.) And within minutes of take-off, as the plane climbed from drizzly gloom to clear sun, I found it's also literally true about light at the end of the tunnel. (I'm not, however, yet ready for *that* tunnel and *that* light. Nor did I particularly want my 'end' on a plane.)

From such experiences when travelling package-class, I now have considerable sympathy for bruised, battered and torn parcels. I know how they feel.

Lesson to be learnt: Think twice before going on a package holiday. Or at least, think about it from the package's point of view.

More political lesson: If you don't have a voice, don't expect any influence.

Lesson for others to learn: To be a successful pusher, you also need brains.

Unfortunately, this was not my worst package experience. Flying to America, I had arranged that my teenage son would help me. (On such a long flight, even an oversized pee-bag one would burst without someone to empty it.) I would meet him at Heathrow; he travelling there by bus; me, by connecting flight. That, anyway was the plan. But the airport pusher knew better. Despite my protestations, he wheeled me away from our arranged meeting point. I tried to speak over my shoulder. He took no notice. I persisted, till, eventually, he reassured me: "Your son will meet you at the other end." I was not reassured. And even less reassured when we boarded a travellator – obviously our journey would be long.

As he obviously didn't understand me – or care – I realized I must write things down. Fortunately, in my pouch, is paper and pencil for just such contingencies. Unfortunately, *on* my pouch was hand-luggage and crutches, to which I had to hold – and the pencil was at the pouch bottom, so necessitating emptying everything out. *And* we were travelling at speed, round bends and up and down ramps. I did eventually manage to get the pencil, but now had to write at nose-level. The resulting illegible message didn't stop my pusher until we got to the bus-stop for another terminal. Now desperate, I threw down my bags and wrote another message. "Your son knows" he wrote back – as it was obvious I was now deaf.

Trains, planes, boats and me

At the other terminal, however: no son, nor anyone knowing anything about what was going on. My pleas ignored, I felt like a totally helpless piece of baggage. This didn't help pre-flight calmness levels. Nor did repeated announcements that unattended baggage would be removed and destroyed. Fortunately, I was always attended, even if by someone who didn't care.

Eventually, we did meet up. So everything was - as usual – alright in the end. In this case, as 'the end' took two and a half hours, it was dangerously near the END.

Lesson to be learnt: Even the most hopeless situations turn out alright in the end.

Further lesson to be learnt: Try to avoid hopeless situations.

Final lesson: Try to avoid the end.

Post-final lesson: All experiences, however bad at the time, are better afterwards. Some, however, may take years to learn to appreciate

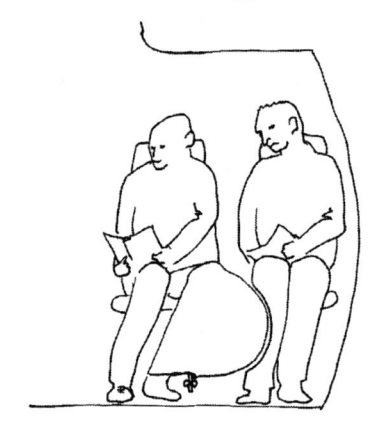

Extra-large pee-bags are extra-discrete for air-travel.

Boat

To go to France for microkinesiolgie therapy, required a ferry crossing from Dover - a new adventure. How I could possibly get out of the car when it was sardine-packed on board ship? I need a lot of space - and not too long a walk - to the passenger decks. A sea-crossing trapped on the car-deck was a daunting prospect.

I needn't have worried, however. Arriving at Dover harbour, my carer asked if disabled passengers could get any special treatment. They could. We were given a special red sign to display and told to drive into an empty waiting-lane. Within minutes an official appeared in front of us, spread his arms and clicked his fingers. Confused, my carer clicked hers back. (She couldn't spread her arms without hitting me in the face. Carers aren't meant to do that.) The official started to make irritated, impatient, movements. This was no help to advance communication.

Clearly frustrated, he came over to the car and signed her to open the window. "Hazard lights." he said, then walked away. I'm quite used to being treated like a package when travelling, but this was the first time I have been treated like a hazardous package. Nonetheless, it had some advantages: we were first aboard, so my fears of no space to get out of the car were groundless.

On board, everything was easy. The boat rocked gently in the harbour swell but, as long as my carer held the wheelchair, this caused no problem. Whenever she let go, however, the wheelchair likewise moved gently from port to starboard and back again.

Beyond the breakwater, however, the significance of this gentle swell became clear. Here, the wind was at gale force and the seas huge. The ship pitched, rolled and occasionally stopped dead with a reverberating hollow clang whenever it slammed into head-waves. My wheelchair wanted to join in the fun. It would have happily cannonballed from side to side if allowed. This would not have been my idea of fun. Fortunately, my carer found an unoccupied bench-seat in the restaurant. (Actually, the restaurant was inexplicably empty.) She helped me lie down. Wedged by the wheelchair (docile now that it didn't have me in it), I couldn't roll off the seat. In this position, the movements of the ship rocked me to sleep. Occasionally, however, I would be wakened by crashes of crockery accompanied by peals of laughter from the kitchen. At such times, I was dimly aware of other passengers hunched over white paper bags, praying. At least, they were kneeling and repeating; "Oh God". For me, however, this was a comfortable night's sleep.

Lesson to be learnt: wheelchairs are good to keep you in place.

Trains

When I started to be disabled, Paddington Station in London used to make me nervous. I would arrive half-an hour before my train was due to depart, but not know which platform I needed. This would only appear on the illuminated boards about five minutes before departure time, namely four minutes before the train doors would be sealed. I never knew if I could walk far enough in four minutes. Added to which was the risk of being pushed over by surging crowds. Another - and totally unpredictable - hazard was panicking runners, who cut through queues at right angles, jumping over feet – far too fast to see crutches. Their only thought was how to catch their train at any price. This price included a trail of tripped-up assorted old ladies and cripples. I hoped I wouldn't be one.

Fortunately, a friend told me about Disabled Assistance. Now all I needed to do was wait in an office and then be collected by an electric cart. True, I had to climb high (which I could then, but can't now). Thereafter, the cart bulldozed its way through the crowds (and suicidal runners) below.

Disabled Assistance always worked perfectly to *leave* Paddington. On the journeys themselves, however, it only *sometimes* worked perfectly. In fact, two times out of five, it didn't work at all. This wasn't always forgetfulness, incompetence, disorganization or not caring. Sometimes the Disabled Assistance Service had a good excuse. At one station, my train arrived late (this does occasionally happen, but only one train in two does so - unless you read the rail company statistics, where it is one train in one hundred). This meant that the office was closed. So what could they do? Of more concern to me was what could *I* do? This wasn't only a problem for me, but for the station staff too. When they locked up the station for the night, I wouldn't be able to walk out. As their insurance company wouldn't allow them to leave me in the unattended station in case I stole it, they would have to put me in a wheelchair to get me out. Fortunately the brightest of them realized that it would be less trouble, and a shorter distance - so less effort - to put me in the same wheelchair to get me to my next train.

Lesson to be learnt: when charity fails, try to encourage intelligence.

Sometimes Disabled Assistance just forgets - after all they're only human. But when they remember - only just in time - they make up for tardiness with enthusiasm. This is not always well directed. To get off trains, I need to give my sticks or crutches to somebody, then grip the handrails and carefully step down. When I reach platform level, my friend is meant to hand me back my sticks. But on one occasion she didn't. She wasn't even there. Speedy with guilt, a man had rushed up with a wheelchair and, seeing her with two sticks, bundled her in and started off. She was too surprised to speak; and I was left hanging on to the train. The guard wanted to get the train away but I, stickless, so with no visual clue as to my disability, was delaying it. He didn't like that. Fortunately I couldn't, or dared not, move - so, like life, everything got sorted out in the end.

There can also be other problems getting off trains. Because I'm so slow disembarking, I always try to arrange my journey to only change trains at a terminating station. I started this when still only on one stick. On one train, however, imagine my horror when, approaching the doors to get out, I heard the 'peep, peep, peep' presaging the doors closing. They not only closed but *locked*. Within seconds the train would be off to a nice quiet siding for its nightly sleep. The doors wouldn't open. With my stick, I pushed the emergency stop button. They still wouldn't open, but in about five minutes the conductor approached. He told me I should be quicker. I tried to explain that one aspect of disability is loss of the ability to run. He was not amused. But neither was I.

There aren't just problems *between* trains, but also *on* them. One small problem - but of major significance to me - is how can I have a pee? This may sound easy enough - a simple matter of bodily function - but hygiene requires it be done in the toilet. How can I get there? At speed, the train is lurching, shaking and swaying. If I hold onto seat headrests, I can possibly - at some risk - work my way slowly along the corridor, but then there are gaps - seats facing the other way or luggage space. Better to wait till the train stops. Unfortunately whenever it stops, a current of people who want to get off flows down the aisle. As I'm slow, I wait till they are past and follow them. But almost immediately comes a reverse current of people who want to get on! Nothing for it but to hold onto a headrest and let them past. But now the train starts up again. I can manage a few more steps before it reaches full lurching speed. Now I must hold on till the next station. This time I'm in the way of people desperately hurrying to catch their connecting trains. If I'm lucky, I can get to the luggage rack, good hand-grips here. If I'm unlucky, somebody wants to take out luggage - some people are so inconsiderate. When I do get to the toilet, I will now have to repeat the whole journey in reverse. At least this time though, I know the 'mountaineering route' - all the handholds.

Nowadays, the Disabled Assistance team seat me near the disabled toilet. This is a shorter journey but, as I'm slower, no less easy. On new trains, this toilet is huge with button-controlled electric doors: one button to open them, one to shut them, one to lock. How many people go into toilets, shut the doors but don't want to lock them? Unfortunately, on all the trains I've been on, a lighted sign outside this toilet said 'out of order'. The light, however, was so weak that I could never be sure if it was on, or if I was just reading a reflection. As it would be impossible to get to any other toilet, the whole carriage length away, I had no choice but to use it, in-order or out. The first time I used such an in-or-out-of-order toilet, everything seemed to work, but I soon discovered what 'out of order' meant: the automatic doors opened automatically at the most inopportune moment. Unfortunately, once the tap is opened, there's no chance of stopping half-way through! I just had to turn away from the door and pretend to be decent.

Lesson to be learnt: once you start a job, it's best to complete it.

Further lesson to be learnt: some people - and things – speak the literal truth: "Disabled Toilet" can mean exactly that.

Nowadays, with leg bags, pee-technique is different. Just as in terrestrial public toilets, there's nowhere low enough to empty the bag into. The only place I can think of, is to stand in the open doorway when the train stops and aim for the gap between train and platform. I'm not quite sure if this is legal. In the toilet is a sign that says: "Do not use toilet in station." (*Why* shouldn't you use the station toilet? Is it because of competition between different privatized companies?) It doesn't say anything about not using the door. True, you don't see many other people using it, but mountaineers routinely use the downwind side of the tent door, so why not trains? (Indeed, on two-day rock-climbs, first-day hazards include climbers above.) Unlike life, there is no notice of forbiddal - so I don't really know what to do.

Lesson to be learnt: always read instructions.

British trains are (more or less) disabled-friendly. Polish trains aren't. Getting on them is a challenge. From a low platform, there are four ladder-steep steps up the side of the train. Fortunately, there are handrails, but by the second step, these were behind my body. This does not help balance. The nearest indoor handrail was on the door. Pulling merely closed it. No help! The other handrail was out of reach. Fortunately (or, though well-intended, unfortunately), someone seized and lifted me to train level. But the train interior, though nice to look into, was too far away to step onto. Nor could I even reach the handrail. Fortunately again, the science of statics and dynamics came to the rescue. Even a strong man can't hold a body-weight at arm's length without overbalancing or taking a step forward. My unknown strong helper was no exception. As he couldn't step into the track, he merely overbalanced, sliding my feet neatly onto the carriage floor. My friend, already on the train, caught me and I was safely aboard.

Lesson to be learnt: While I *always* appreciate help, it's *always* better if helpers understand how to do things.

Now came the problem of moving along the train. The corridor was too narrow to use crutches, and there were no handrails. I looked around. Rock-climbing time again. First handhold: a door handle, in easy reach. This, however, opened the door to the toilet - not my destination. Next handhold - quite high up: a green handle (or was it red? That's the problem with being colour-blind.) Unfortunately, though I thought it was just within reach, my friend didn't let me try. Beyond these, there was only the window gasket and a few rivet-heads - neither much use. Fortunately, the train waited the five minutes it took to shuffle to the nearest compartment where someone kindly gave up a seat for me. This was all relatively safe - in retrospect. Not so getting off!

Our destination station, being on the tourist map, was better quality, hence had higher platforms. This meant less height down, but a wider gap - about twice as far as I can step. I didn't relish the thought of falling between platform and train. It's not nice down there. (I know: some twelve years previously, I had slid down there to rescue a child. Lots of electrical cables, grease and only a narrow gap to get out of. The child got lots of attention - so much there was nobody to help me get out; this took twenty minutes!)

I descended the two steps to platform level - but what now? At this point, a well-meaning stranger reached over, grabbed my arms and pulled. I fell forward and he tottered backwards, his arched back ensuring my body leant forwards so my feet were high. True: it was a bit undignified, but getting there was more important than *how* I got there. Even more important, however, would be getting back.

Now we knew what to do, the return journey should have been much safer. No insuperable gap problems when de-training, just a long, careful descent. I had, however, reckoned without the conductor. If I fell, it would be his responsibility. If the train was delayed, this also would be his responsibility.

Trains, planes, boats and me

Which would be worse? In fact, as both were likely, he would be doubly responsible. Poor man! Standing on the platform below, he was visibly shaking with worry. Also, he was neither big nor strong, but clearly felt he had to act as though he was. While I was reaching for handholds so I could turn for a ladder-wise descent, he pulled my hands down. Naturally, I lost my balance. Fortunately, my friend grabbed me from above. This slowed descent sufficiently for me to step down twice. I was now at her full stretch, so the conductor pulled again. Again I fell uncontrollably, this time onto his neck - to which I held on hard. Very undignified for him - but (slightly) safer for me. Unfortunately, his angle of pull jammed my heel under the step above. I feared his pull (or collapse under my weight) would break my ankle. Fortunately again, though unable to speak - I was able to stop him and extricate my foot. By now, other pairs of hands were sharing the load and I arrived at the platform and straight into my wheelchair. I'm not sure who was the more relieved: the conductor or me.

Lesson to be learnt: Enthusiasm gets things done. Indeed, it's indispensable. But only with understanding can things be done safely.

Further lesson to be learnt: Teamwork can work miracles. But it needs a miracle for non-teamwork to work.

Final lesson: Life isn't *always* fun - at the time. But it can be funny afterwards. This is good because, as death comes after life, even if living isn't always fun, dying can be.

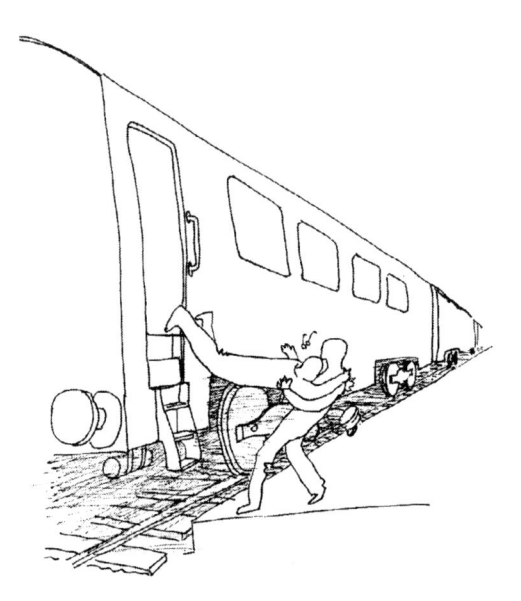

Disabled disembarking.

22. Cars and their drivers

All sorts of Cars

I never used to think about getting into cars. Now I have to use technique. This is preferable to 'learning from mistakes' – which sometimes hurt! My own car is quite straightforward. Anyway, once I've succeeded in opening the self-closing door without losing my balance, it is. All I now need do is throw my crutches in, disentangle them from the handbrake, throw them in again, get them off my seat and onto the passenger's, disentangle them from the handbrake again.... This would be easy to sort out when sitting - but, until sorted out, it's impossible to sit.

Crutches eventually parked, I now (try to) get in. With one hand, I hold the door-handle, with the other the steering wheel. Now I must get my left foot in (less straightforward), and - if possible, in a controlled manner - sit down while not pulling the steering wheel off. At this point, if someone is helping me, they usually say: "Watch your head!" but as I can't see my head, I never know how to watch it. Next, I must get my right foot in. Now all I have to do is, without falling out, lean just beyond my reach to get one finger tip on the door-handle, then two finger tips, then three, eventually four, and so shut the door. I now need to fish the safety belt out of narrow slot between seat and door. This usually necessitates opening the door, which then often catches the wind and swings wide. I now reach for the door again, again trying not to fall out. But this time, being loosely strapped in, I wouldn't fall the whole way but would end up suspended with my face several inches above the ground. With no body-ground contact, this doesn't count as a fall - so that's alright. Nonetheless, this is not a good position for driving a car. All this is relatively easy, namely easily takes twenty minutes.

Would this be easier were I passenger, not driver? Unfortunately, the passenger side is less easy. Inconsiderately, there is no steering wheel on that side. This only leaves the door for my left hand to hold, and the door-frame for my right. My car is a respectable dark colour - part of my (mostly failed) attempt to be respectable. This is relevant: it means that on hot sunny days the metal is hot and I burn my fingers. Nevertheless, like abseiling, it is rather important to hold on! Next I try to raise my right foot enough to get it in. It isn't very willing, lazy foot. After several attempts it usually does get in, or at least, half-in - it must, because if it doesn't I am stuck. Then all I have to do is put my right elbow on the windscreen so I'm holding the door-frame with my armpit (in lieu of a third hand), slide carefully down while at the same time swinging my body so as to sit on the edge of the seat. But this is a precision maneuver: Not armpit-grip too tightly so I jam, nor too loosely so I fall away from the car. Also, I mustn't swing so far I bang my head, nor so little I miss the seat and sit on the ground. This would be a mistake. Indeed the only bit of me in the right place would be my right foot, now above my head, and so not very useful. With practice, I usually do this right.

Other sorts of cars require different techniques. For Landrovers, I hold the dashboard handle and seat belt (doubled, this won't slip). I now get first my left foot, then my right, onto the step. Next, I must get my left foot up to the cab floor. Then comes the difficult bit: I need a new right hand-hold. The seat edge is nearest but my hand can easily slip off that. Having proved this by experiment, I don't feel the need to prove it again. It is an alarmingly long way to the ground. Sometimes, therefore, I open the tool-box and grasp its lip. This is a good hand-hold, so the right thing to do - if all goes well. If, however, I fail to get my right foot past my left, I'm now left listing at about forty-five degrees. This is an uncorrectable list and as I can't hold on for long, there are only two options: I can either slide out - this would be painful - or lower myself gently in. This is painless but it inserts my face into the toolbox, leaving my throat supported by its edge. This is uncomfortable. Moreover, the view is dull. From this position, all I can do is wriggle. This changes nothing, but does look ridiculous so it's hard not to laugh. Laughing into tools while employing a rock-climbing throat-hold has interesting acoustic effects. This also changes nothing. It does, however, help to pass the time.

Lesson to be learnt: some parts of cars aren't fun to look at - anyway, not for too long.

Little Cars

In small rooms, it's easy to find a wall to plant my crutches against to reduce slip risk. Also there is always something to hold onto, lean against or – at worst - fall on at half velocity, after which it's only another half velocity to the floor. This is twice as good (or, anyway: half as bad) as hitting the floor at full velocity. With my disability, this makes small safer and easier than big.

Not so with cars. The smallest car I've ever been in was a Polish 'Maluch'. So small are these that, stood on end, four would fit in an average bedroom – still leaving room for the bed. (Why anyone would want four vertical cars in their bedroom is beyond me. Indeed, I can't even understand why anyone would want to sleep in a vertical bed!)

Getting in (to the car, not bed) wasn't easy. It's not that Poles are small, but clearly they are more agile than me. To start with, the door only opens thirty degrees. As my technique is to stand on one foot while putting the other in the car, I must therefore stand level with the seat back (perhaps Poles do something different with feet so they don't need to stand on one?) This means I am completely out of balance. As long as I hold the ceiling handle, it's quite safe - I won't fall out. Indeed I can even lower myself so a quarter of my bottom is on the seat. There's no chance to swing my body in – I would hit my neck on the doorframe. So long as I hold on, this is still safe but it's not the optimum for travelling, even were I able to borrow a skateboard for the foot left out in the cold. Fortunately, my friend has always helped me at this stage.

Nor are these safe cars to break down in. At night, first the lights went out, then, approaching a railway level crossing, the engine cut out and the car glided to rest – by good fortune, fifty yards beyond it. We were now half on the verge, half on the road. Rush hour traffic screeched, roared and thundered past us. (And this in a country whose drivers are famous as organ-donors.) Being disabled, I was stuck in the car. Not so my friend; I therefore ordered her out. She refused. One disadvantage of disability is that I couldn't throw her out, so we could only sit, pretending to be safe, and wait for a friend with a towrope. In that forty minutes only one car stopped. A car full of women, so I was impressed. All they wanted to do, however, under the pretext of asking the way, was to see what was going on. (Apparently, interesting things can happen when a man and a woman share a parked car – even half-on a busy road.) Dissapointed, they drove off without helping.

I should have learnt long ago that fear doesn't help anybody. (My neighbourhood wasp tried to teach me this for years.) Once I've done all I can do - in this case: nothing – what will or won't happen, will or won't. There's nothing more I can do about it, so why waste energy worrying? The worst that could happen is that I'll end up dead, but this is probably going to happen one day anyway. True: it may not exactly be fun, but it's more relaxing to sit for forty minutes not-worrying than worrying. This however, is no protection against cold. This made me a bit nervous about catching a cold. Little old cars – especially crippled ones – are clearly a health-risk.

Lesson to be learnt: Danger may be unavoidable, but try to keep warm – it feels nicer.

Big Cars

Big cars are easier - anyway in theory. A roof rack rail is great to hold onto but once my feet are in the car, this does leave me swinging outside. Transfer to seat-back handholds involves delicate maneuvers. Once again I am glad of my rock climbing experience.

Lesson to be learnt: Don't be fooled by grandeur.

Even Bigger Cars

American cars, even small ones, are larger – and more luxurious – than large European cars. Correspondingly higher, they offer commanding views. But with the floor too high to step up to, how could I get in? Fortunately my son came to the rescue. He lifted me under the armpits, dragged me up and dumped me in the seat. This solved the problem of getting me in, and made it possible to get to an important design meeting. Unfortunately, however, it did not get my trousers in. When I was dragged over the seat edge, they weren't. In fact they were pushed down. Trousers may not be essential for commanding views, but for client meetings, they do add dignity. To compensate for my inability to speak, this – and trousers - are essential.

Lesson to be learnt: A commanding position can – and hopefully does – conceal deficiencies below.

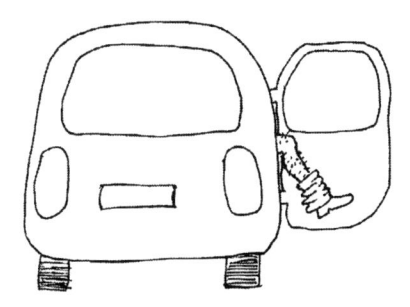

Some cars require ignominious boarding technique.

Disabled Taxis

Disabled Taxis can be quite disabling or, at least, disempowering. They're built to winch in, or hoist, wheelchair and occupant. But I don't want to sit like an isolated package in the back. I would rather sit with friends and enjoy the view from a normal height seat. Usually, this is (perhaps grudgingly) acceptable, but one driver was definitely not amused – why couldn't I be winched in like an obedient package? To get to a proper seat I had to climb up two high steps. There was a handle on the doorpost, though mounted too close for a whole hand to fit in, only fingertips. But what could be the next handhold? The seat backs were smooth and rounded; also they moved. But there was nothing else to hold. Sure enough the seat tipped back, my hand slipped off and I swung from three fingertips. As these were now behind my feet this swung me out and nearly onto my back some distance below. Fortunately a policeman was reprimanding the taxi driver for parking and he caught me. So the driver enjoyed the pleasure of being right, I avoided time in hospital and the policeman did his good deed for the day. This made everybody happy.

Cars and their drivers

Lesson to be learnt: For (continuing) life, balance is even more important than three-point support.

Additional lesson to be learnt: If expecting to be treated like a package, expect a system designed to make me behave like one.

All-Terrain Vehicles

All-terrain vehicles are the ultimate for disabled travel. But they aren't all-terrain. I should, of course, have learnt this from 100% grape-juice. Contents: aqua, sugar, fructose, sucrose, saccharine, citric acid, flavorings, preservative, 100% grape-juice. Recyclable container. (I didn't know I was expected to drink this too!)

When designing a school in America, I rode in one - a sort-of electric tractor-and-cart - to inspect the site. Utilitarian but fast. My fifteen-year old son drove. This was fun – for him. I was more concerned about what to do if – as seemed inevitable at that speed - it turned over. Miraculously, we survived the day. In the evening, however, twenty-seven of the twenty-eight teachers went home, and one offered to drive me round the forest backing the site. Unfortunately, the narrow path led over a boulder. Could we get over it? My driver inched the vehicle forward. Yes! The front-axel cleared it easily. But the rear-axel never got a go. Halfway across, we grounded and ended up with all four wheels in the air. At this point the vehicle ceased being all-terrain. I did, however, half learn how gnomes feel when sitting on toadstools. (*Half* learn because I didn't have a fishing rod to complete the experience.)

But what to do now? Our chariot wouldn't accelerate off, rock off or slide off – and everyone else had gone home. Worse, it would soon become dark. And worse again, it would soon be mosquito supper-time. I suggested levering it off with a stick. As I couldn't speak, I drew a picture. But I only drew one stick. In the event, this immediately broke into two. Mosquito supper-time was now even nearer. Fortunately my driver was a burly man. (Doubly fortunate as this would give the mosquitoes more supper, lessening their demands on me.) He lifted me bodily out the seat and laid me against a tree. He and my son now managed to tip the vehicle till its rear wheels touched the ground. He then leant over and pressed the accelerator with a stick. Through the mud-spray directed at my face, I saw the vehicle leap backwards onto another rock. This one, however, didn't hold it fast, so we could re-board and reverse half-a-mile through dense, and now twilit, trees, arriving at our car exactly as the mosquito-supper-buzzer sounded.

Lessons to be learnt: don't believe everything you read. Don't recycle 100% grape-juice. Don't all-terrainize all-terrain vehicles. Don't feed the mosquitoes – however much they sing for their supper. And definitely don't drink containers.

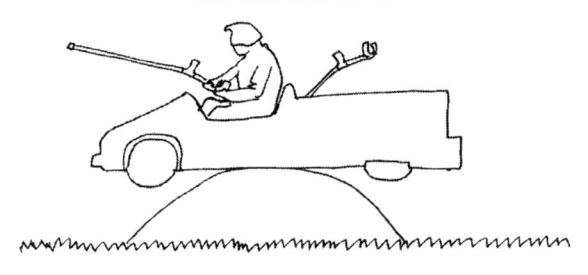

Gnome-on-mushroom practice.

Drivers

I may not be able to walk well, but I at least I can drive. Am I safe? Generally teenagers are convinced I am not. I'm not convinced they are. I can't fall over when I'm driving so that makes it safe for me. Is it safe for other road users? My foot reaction is slow – about half a second from accelerator to brake. Cars travel far in half a second, but I argue that my anticipation is many seconds ahead of teenagers' and my speed allows leisured braking. Theirs doesn't.

I don't drive long distances, nor on fast roads. For such things I need drivers. Some are good, some are safe, and some are 'interesting'.

There are cultural aspects to driving. One American driver had learnt that in any dangerous situation you should always accelerate. This may make sense on Californian Freeways but I never found it calmed my nerves. Whenever someone (including her) did something wrong, she would shout "Hello" and make hand gestures. Obviously Californian driving is based on friendship to strangers.

Lesson to be learnt: Always extend the hand of friendship (being careful not to extend the wrong fingers) – even to idiots. If something has been their fault, that is good – I know I'm not to blame. If it has been mine – that too is good: I can't bear them any resentment. If we have both been to fault…. Well, that's how it is in life.

There are also psychological aspects. These, I discovered, were particularly pronounced in a psychiatrist's driving. On one occasion, seeking a guesthouse after a lecture we discovered nobody knew where it was. I had been taken there by taxi – from somewhere else the night before: no help! We did have a map: local footpaths. This showed roads but not priorities nor the sweeps that traffic engineers use to turn a right-angled T-junction into an uninterruptedly flowing road. Hence we failed to recognize many turnings. Also our destination village wasn't on the map – only the 'nether' version; ours was the 'major'. None of this helped harmony. After a long fruitless search, the driver remembered he had the phone number. He phoned for directions and was told "straight on about half a mile." After five miles, it became obvious that he had omitted to ask which way the car should be facing. These were not an uneventful five miles. Whenever we passed a group of houses he would ask if I recognized the

Cars and their drivers

guesthouse. I didn't and he became increasingly irritated. I had stayed there so why didn't I recognize it? How could I? It wasn't the house. Finally we tried driving the other way. Sure enough, after five and a half miles, there it was. As I opened the door to get out I saw a real, large-scale map in the door pocket. But, after all, the driver *was* a psychiatrist.

There can also be physiological, or at least, medical issues: One driver-cum-odd-job man couldn't help going to sleep. This was never a problem when doing jobs oddly, but it was whenever he drove me somewhere. Initially, I thought the desperate increase in speed, zigzagging and late cornering were just bad driving. Later I came to realize he was racing against his closing eyes. But I only learnt this on the Day of the Near Miss. When we went straight round a bend – namely: across the road towards an oncoming car, I did wonder if this was a safe way to drive. My speech and movements are slow, so by the time I had taken a breath, opened my mouth and got my tongue to work - it takes some reminding, lazy thing - he had woken up. This was fortunate or I would have never finished this book. What a waste of work it would have been to only write half a book. We passed quite (namely: very!) close to the other driver and I noticed that he had an unhealthy white complexion. Perhaps he was, or thought he might be just about to be, on the way to hospital.

Lesson to be learnt: life is good. I'd like more of it.

There can also be communication issues. One driver was excellent, careful, competent and with a comfortable car. But his hearing was poor and, in particular, he was deaf in the left ear. My speech is bad and, when I twist to the right, also particularly weak. In British cars I sit on the left, the driver on the right. Not a good combination.

The first part of the journey I knew, but - from the route we went - he didn't. As there was much grumbling about small roads (which I had always thought were large) I deemed it wise to keep quiet. The middle part neither of us knew – another good reason to be quiet. But the last part I knew and he didn't. Hence I felt I should tell him the way. This was not a good idea.

"Take the next left." "You need to stop for a pee?" "No – next left!" "We'll stop in the next lay-by." "Take the next right turn and turn around, we've just missed our turn." "You've just pissed? I hope you didn't wet the seat!" Clearly time to stop talking and when we eventually got to the lay-by, try to communicate by drawing a map - a map of what *I* wanted to say, not of what *he* thought I had done.

Lesson to be learnt: let other people do things their way. As they like to know that they are right, it is better not to disagree, just pee in the right places.

At Work

23. Conferences

Working from home is relatively straightforward. Conferences (relatively) aren't. In theory, I just go there to sit and listen, possibly speak. In theory also, a friend or helper can wheel me to the right place to sit. It is then my responsibility to listen. I'm good at this - when the talk is interesting enough to listen to. But it's only human to have lapses, and being ill I have a perfect excuse for even more lapses whenever things are boring. No problem here. If I nod off, or even snore, everybody knows (I hope) that I'm just having balance or breathing difficulties.

Problems, however, start with wheelchairs.

In theory - and normally in practice - I am wheeled to the right place at the right time. But theories say nothing about being wheeled back. Usually, there are main lectures - where we all sit together - and smaller workshops where we don't. At one conference, the workshops were in seminar rooms opening off a ramp which spiralled around the main auditorium. My friend took great care to push me to the workshop of my choice before going to his.

But how to get back? I wheel myself slowly and, my left arm being weaker than my right, in left-handed curves. Not to hold everybody up, I therefore waited to leave the seminar room till everyone, except those lingering in conversation, had. To reach the door would require several reverses and pivots on the spot. There was also a ramp up to it, fortunately not too steep even for my weak arms. It would, in fact, have been (relatively) easily manageable had I gone straight up. But I didn't. I swung left. With a weak left arm, this was predictable and initially no problem. When I started to graze the wall, however, it was clearly time to straighten up. Straightening up meant a short reverse. Aided by gravity, this brought me back to the foot of the ramp. Several attempts and I got no further. Some people, late for the next event, slipped by me but, to ask for help, I could only speak to the back of their heads. Not knowing their names, my weak voice couldn't attract attention. Nor could I turn my body to address anyone else before they became back-of-heads. Eventually someone noticed my predicament and wheeled me through the door to the level landing outside. He then rushed off, so becoming yet another back-of-head. Being slow to speak, he was out of earshot by the time I managed to ask for further help.

But now a bigger challenge loomed: the downhill ramp. This had been built in the days when 1:12 ramps were permitted. (Nowadays only a sissy 1:18 is allowed.) Coming from a country where 1:4 roads aren't uncommon (1:4 on the *outside* of the bend. The inside of the bend, being shorter, is steeper: usually 1:1.),

Conferences

1:12 sounds almost horizontal. But, one floor up, in a wheelchair with brakes that, even when parked, won't hold on a slope, it feels vertiginously steep. Could I dare a semi-controlled descent? *Semi*-controlled because the first yard would probably be controllable, the rest not. To make matters worse, every so often, doors near the bottom would open and unsuspecting pedestrians crossed the about-to-be bobsleigh run. Moreover, my weak voice was useless for shouting warnings. And despite the wheelchair's rapid acceleration capabilities, as well as (effectively) no brakes, it had no horn.

Fortunately, after some five minutes indecision, someone noticed me and came to the rescue.

Lesson to be learnt: it's not always so bad to be slow. Speed kills.

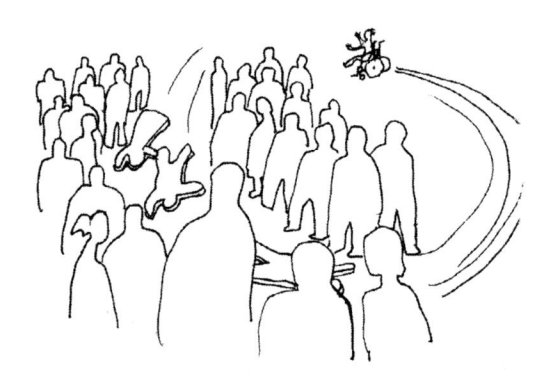

Ramps are good – especially for wheelchair-bobsleigh (or slaying anybody else).

Conference lectures are (more or less) manageable, but at conferences I also need to pee. This isn't always so easy. There are the usual disabled-accessible but leg-bag-inaccessible toilets - no help to me. At this conference, the only leg-bag accessible toilet was the tree outside. Here I spent many botanical visits, apparently (I hoped) studying the insect life at its roots, but actually feeling more like a dog marking its territory.

At another conference, all forty-two participants would sit in a circle to discuss the lecture theme. At tea-breaks there would be the usual rush to queue for the toilet. But I, with catheter and leg-bag, enjoyed location-independence, so circle-time seemed as good a pee-time as any. Unfortunately, the participants were polite. Each waited for the preceding speaker to finish. In the intervening pause, my plumbing gurgle broke the hush. Embarrassing. I tried to interrupt the flow till someone else started to speak. But then my foot began to feel warm. In the cool weather, this initially felt quite pleasant - until I started to wonder *why* it was warm. Why just *one* foot? Why the foot with the leg-bag? Could the tap be open? Hasty calculations: what is the cubic capacity of a size nine shoe? What is the volume of a foot? Subtract latter from former. How many cups of tea had

Conferences

I drunk that morning? What volume of liquid did these add up to? How long before a telltale overflow would snake across the floor towards the centre of the circle? Its origin - and what it was (obviously not spilt tea) - would be unequivocal. No chance to evade responsibility by blaming the dog. This was the best cure for incontinence I've ever encountered.

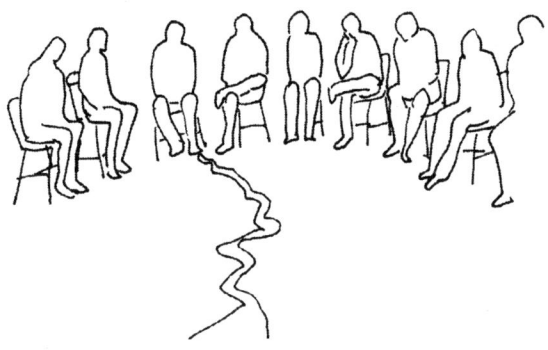

It wasn't me.

Not all conferences are in disabled-friendly locations. One, in particular, had its lecture venue upstairs. Access was by an external stone staircase. This had an iron handrail, so the ascent, though slow, was (more or less) safe. Once at the top, transfer from handrail to non-handrail landing was less safe. Going down, however, was another story.

I didn't feel at all safe poised on the cliff edge, mentally preparing myself for the transfer move from crutches to handrail. This would have been bad enough when dry. But it never was. With my slow, ultra-cautious, descent, I would be totally rain soaked by the time I reached the bottom. Fortunately (?), like unavoidably walking through puddles instead of stepping over them, I am used to that by now. When you're disabled, there are some things you just have to live with! Worse than that, everything was a bit slippery, making it only just (in other words: almost) safe. Living with being wet is one thing, but I didn't want to have to die with this. The rain-puddled landing felt like an ice-sheeted cliff edge. Nonetheless, there was nothing for it but to try. With great caution, I edged towards the yawning lip. But here, other conference participants came to the rescue. Two strong men seized me and forced my arms over their shoulders. My locked shoulder-joint obliged, but not without pain. This caused the arm to go limp so I couldn't hold on and needed even more faith in destiny than usual. They then picked up my legs and leaped down the steps. Their confident leap quickly deteriorated into an unconfident stagger as they discovered they needed technique and safety training, but unfortunately (and especially unfortunate for me) had neither.

Conferences

All three of us having (by the grace of God) arrived safely at the bottom, they finished with a flourish by loading me feet first into a car. Feet in car, but arms over some two bodies' shoulders outside the car isn't ideal for balance. In fact, it's actually a rather difficult position to get into a car from, but nobody had thought of that. The foot-half of me was safe, but not the head-half. Nor was it dry. Eventually, but not without knocking one pair of glasses off, they got me in. Such fun did this look (to anyone outside the operation) and so much laughter, that others wanted to try it. Over the week, I was carried by progressively weaker men with poorer balance and less coordinated feet. This convinced me that no conference should last longer than one week.

This flying technique proved to have other applications. When we went on a mountain outing, the plan was to drive in Landrovers as far as possible, then walk. But what about me? I would have to stay behind in the parked vehicle. Fortunately, I didn't have to, but was seized by enthusiastic hands and borne aloft. Unfortunately, however, the hill was steeper than it looked, so before long my bearers were staggering. But, short of dropping me in the mud, what could they do? Fortunately, others came to the rescue. As I was now carried by relays, nobody needed to choose between loss of male prestige and heart attack.

But then it began to rain. Being in Scotland and on a mountain, 'rain' is an understatement. This was a solid wall of water driven horizontally. Someone did up my coat so water would run off me, but down my bearers' necks. At this point, the army came to the rescue. They had provided one Landrover and driver to help get us to the start of the walk, no further. But here it now came, bounding over the rough ground. Gratefully, my bearers loaded me aboard. Being driven, however, proved even more adventurous than being carried. The vehicle pitched, rolled, jerked, shied and slid. The enthusiastic driver assured us it was (almost) quite safe, as we were (so far) always at least (or nearly) five degrees short of the roll point. He went on to describe his war adventures in Iraq. Compared with these, I understood how he could describe our steeplechase journey as safe. I was particularly struck by his compassion for the Iraqis. He recounted how, sent to arrest looters, when the British troops saw their poverty, they were careful to let them get away. This journey made me totally revise my judgmental preconceptions of squaddies.

Lesson to be learnt: Never judge by appearances – even if camouflaged.

Further lesson to be learnt: Justice is blind. So is judgment.

Another conference outing, though listed as a driving tour - which would have suited me - proved to include 'short' walks. These didn't. As the two tour leaders (fortunately in different cars) were constantly criticizing each other, each tried to outdo the other in length of walk. They also competed in roughness of terrain. This didn't help me greatly, as my wheelchair is not an all-terrain one. Here, there was no army, so my friend, the wheelchair and I ended up abandoned

Conferences

at a beauty spot. Beautiful or not, in the rain, mist and midges, we could only christen it 'Midge-view Lake', and divide our time between playing hide and sheep (count sheep visible through mist) and devising tourist-board slogans like: " Home of the Happy Midge" and "Midge Society welcomes tourists".

Lesson to be learnt: beauty is only skin deep. As midges bite skin-deep, where does that leave beauty?

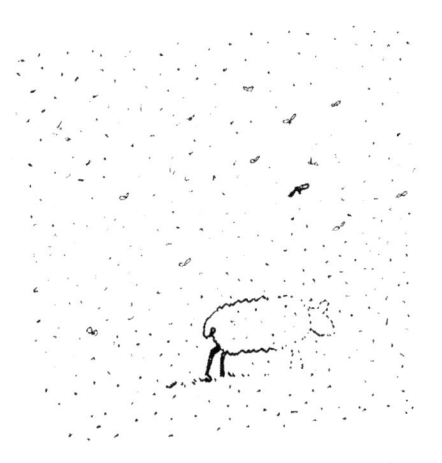

Hide and Sheep at Midge-view Lake.

Life in General, Death in particular

24. Disabled Love

Life has taught me not to believe in love. After these lessons - many and bitter - I knew I would never, could never, fall in love again. But life defies prediction. It brings hope in the most hopeless situations, light in the darkest places and love when everything says it isn't possible. But disabled love isn't easy. Loving is about giving; giving more, much more, than you receive.

It has taken me a lifetime to come to realize this, but now there's not much I can give, certainly almost nothing I can *do* for my beloved. Indeed, I first realized my feelings when I *couldn't* do something for her. She was obviously exhausted and I thought " How nice to wake up after a rest to a cup of tea." (Who would have thought tea could be so romantic?) But there was no way I could make her tea - and this hurt.

Disability means needing things done for me. But need is not a good basis for love. It doesn't leave the other person free; the needy one isn't whole and balanced; and it's a taking, not a giving, gesture. When disabled, it is painfully hard to find ways to give in *deed*, not just in *word*. Words are easy enough - though, in my case, with slurred and difficult speech, even words are hard. Fortunately, as my words aren't easy to understand, she only understands them to be good. This reminds me of healthier times, lecturing in Russia. I could say what I wanted; and the translator say what the audience wanted to hear. This made everybody happy. But words without deeds are empty - facile to say but not backed up by will, so no commitment substance. I've found a few, cruelly few, things I can do: mainly just to be present during life's stressful moments.

It's easy for romance to blossom in romantic situations - easy for most people. I, however, have unromantic habits. Sudden unpredictable food-jetting can spoil any intimate moment. Not the best start! I do try, of course. Naturally I try not to belch while whispering in her ear - or, at least, to keep the belch dry.

Falling in love is a gift. But living in love is work. However flourishing the romantic stage, for love to mean something, to endure, means sharing hardships, angers, stresses, each other's weaknesses and less attractive sides - including, sometimes, half-digested food. It means sharing the full spectrum of life - especially all the things that go wrong. Of these, I have many.

Disability means coming to terms with not being able to *do* things for the one you love. You can only *be* for them. Up till now, my whole giving identity depended on *doing* things. I never had confidence in the value of my *self*. Now this self is all I can give, so I have to work doubly hard to make that self worthy of value. As for things I *can* do: make odd noises, dribble, eat messily, spray food - not all of this is something anyone would want to share.

What unexpected happiness, reasons to live, life brings. What unexpected eyes love opens. What unexpected gifts disability brings.

25. Why Me? Life isn't Fair

Life sometimes feels so unfair. Why me? Why should I be ill?

This is very satisfying as a statement of complaint, but much less so as a question. Simple questions tend to have complicated answers. Why *not* me: should somebody else have my illness?

I've looked around my circle of friends, not-friends and even definitely-not-friends and I can't find anyone I wish to be ill. (If I could, I would have to join that club that turns crosses upside down and does weird things in churchyards at midnight. This wouldn't suit me. I'm so clumsy I would be sure to fall into a grave. Churchyards at night may be alright for the living dead, but they aren't safe for the nearly dead. And anyway I've had enough weird food to put me off weirdos, weirdists and weirdism.)

But, friends, not-friends, definitely-not-friends and strangers, there are many worse off than me. People in pain, in terrifying debt, in crippling poverty, in jobs, relationships, company and places that drain them of energy, people with worries about loved ones or overburdened with depression.

I'm not in pain (falls and therapies excepted). I'm not depressed. I don't have a dead end job. True: life may come to a dead end. What life won't? But does dead end mean end? The evidence of amateur (namely: failed) die-ers suggests not. Furthermore, I don't have anything to worry about - anyway if I did I wouldn't be able to do it, so what is the point of worrying? Also, despite often disastrous income, I've never starved. This actually is not quite as good as it sounds. With one cook, a starvation fast might have been the healthier and tastier option.

Would I prefer an easier, more prosperous life? Of course. On second thoughts though, I'm not so sure. Luxury is a questionable boon in the animal kingdom. On the farm, bulls are pampered, but after two years (a full, and no doubt pleasurable, round of cows) they're sold. After only a few rounds more, they suddenly become beef. Amongst insects, drone bees enjoy every luxury and don't lift a wing to any work. Come autumn, they're turned out to freeze to death. In pre-history also, the Fisher King was indulged with every pleasure (especially the queen) but after a year found himself as a sacrifice. Even nowadays, an awful lot of rich people don't look particularly happy. Some are so busy keeping rich, they aren't even able to laugh at me. Indeed, it's not unknown for millionaires to step off yachts or out of high windows. (They step out of low windows too – risking banging their heads - also *onto* yachts, but these are less newsworthy events.)

For them, however rich, however miserable, just as for me, life isn't fair, things go wrong. Indeed, I have yet to find *anyone* to whom life isn't *un*fair. There are no two ways of looking at it: *Life just isn't fair*. This is a fact. But there are two very opposite conclusions that can be drawn from this: One is that everything goes wrong - how disastrous! Life is constantly, consistently, unfair and worrying. It must be pre-destined to be miserable. The other: that not-fairness, things going wrong, is what life is all about. This makes it exciting, stimulating and fun. It ensures that life just can't be taken too seriously! After all, how boring it would be if everything were easy! Fortunately, it isn't. Anyway, not for me.

Both views are true: Life *is* unfair, and it *is* fun. But we can't *feel* both attitudes at the same time. So it's up to us to chose our viewpoint. For myself, I've had enough of pain, worry, unfairness and burden. I also don't feel like being a victim. I would much rather be a beneficiary. However unpredictable life invariably is, at least I would be in control of the consequences of living, rather than be at their mercy - of which they have none. The fact is: Life as fun is much more fun!

If we view life as a journey of inner growth, what helps us grow? In my experience, it is only through challenge that I have ever managed to learn anything. Only through hardship and pain have I grown. Children are so drawn to adventure because they *need to grow*. Perhaps my problem is that I just haven't grown up. Not that everything in life needs to be adventurous. That could even be a little bit stressful, even compromise life-expectancy.

One curious aspect of things going wrong is: do they? It's been my experience that *everything* works out for *the best* in the end. But 'the best' is often the hardest, so only visible as best after many years. Life has consistently proven this.

Oddly (or not), nobody laughs when things go right. Humour is fed by the odd and unexpected, by things going wrong. And through humour, things going wrong enrich, rather than impoverish, life. Before I was ill, only *some* things would go wrong. This could be extremely irritating. Now, however, *everything* goes wrong. Too much to be irritating! Indeed, it (mostly) makes life funny. As it is only humour that can make sense of life, life would be just a pointless tragedy if it wasn't funny. That was poor Hamlet's big mistake - he took life (and death) too seriously. No wonder Shakespeare needed to write a few comedies after that!

Perhaps indeed, there is a good reason things go wrong in life. Certainly, a life where everything went right wouldn't just be boring, but stultifying. In fact it wouldn't be life.

If life makes any sense, so must dying, for it will almost (?) certainly be part of every life. Life is a terminal condition; we're all dying – some faster than others. Anyone, therefore, who feels miserable about dying, must feel miserable about living. If living is that bad, it must be doubly miserable to feel miserable about dying. (This makes it trebly miserable – which is just *too* bad!) But if you're open to living (and hence, unavoidably, dying) being fun, it *is* fun. This is not to say that everything is *perfect*. It isn't – but that's life! (or, in this case, death.) But my life is certainly better than it was before I became ill.

But does life need to be *quite* so unfair? Must *quite* so many things go wrong? Is that really the only way to make life fun? Do I really have to be ill, just to stop

Why Me? Life isn't Fair

life being boring? This leads to the question: *why* am I ill? I've often wondered, indeed, thought myself into ever-decreasing circles about this. If it's a genetic reason, why didn't my grandparents get it? If it's environmental or dietary, why did I bother to live a healthy life? If it's stress-related, why don't many more people get it? The fact is: it isn't logical. (But why should it be? I'm not a car, nor any other kind of machine, but an illogical being.) There's absolutely no way to make sense of it. The plain fact is: Life's a bummer – absolutely *not* fair. When you're down it kicks you in the teeth. I learnt this at least as far back as my student days: when I had a hangover, my face looked awful too. But only more recently did I learn the *lesson*: When you're *up*, life is good to you. This, however, still does nothing to explain why I have to be ill. It's nothing to do with keeping up, down or sideways. All this thinking is exhausting, dispiriting and gets me nowhere fast.

But is it so bad to be ill? Or could it, in fact, be a blessing? Do blessings come by chance? If so, there's always hope. But personally, I no longer believe in chance. Far from making life hopeless, however, if things *don't* happen by chance, this unavoidably must change my outlook on illness, on dying – indeed on everything.

What if I started at the other end: what has my illness *given* to me?

Incapacity has come on slowly, and early on I definitely didn't enjoy it. Initially limping was embarrassing, falls in public even more so. But time after time, closed-faced strangers would help me - and as they helped, their faces opened. I realised that some had not had a chance to help someone all day, all week, perhaps all year. My incapacity was a gift to them.

It has also been a gift to me. There are so many things I can't do – so there go a whole package of worries. Anyway some - like washing up – I never enjoyed anyway. There goes another package of drudgery. And what I can do, I usually do wrong. I also make odd sounds, dribble, spill food and am generally embarrassing. But life's too short to be embarrassed *all* the time. So I end up finding it funny. Unfortunately, if something's funny I can't help laughing. Fortunately, once I start to laugh it seems (nearly) everybody else does too. *Nearly* everyone – some few think I'm half-witted, mad or odd. They may well be right, but if they are steadfastly, stiffly, not amused, that is *their* problem - not mine. Their problem because frankly, life *is* funny. I never knew this when I was healthy; I had to become ill to find that out.

Could this be the answer to my original question? Could it possibly be that I *needed* to become ill, to enjoy life? That dying helped me discover that life is fun. Anyway, it seems that (my) dying is fun.

26. Last words

If you enjoyed this book, you may be interested in the sequel: *Dying **was** Fun*. (Look for it in the '**Death**'☠ section of your local bookstore.) Unfortunately, as paper burns, I haven't yet worked out how to write this.

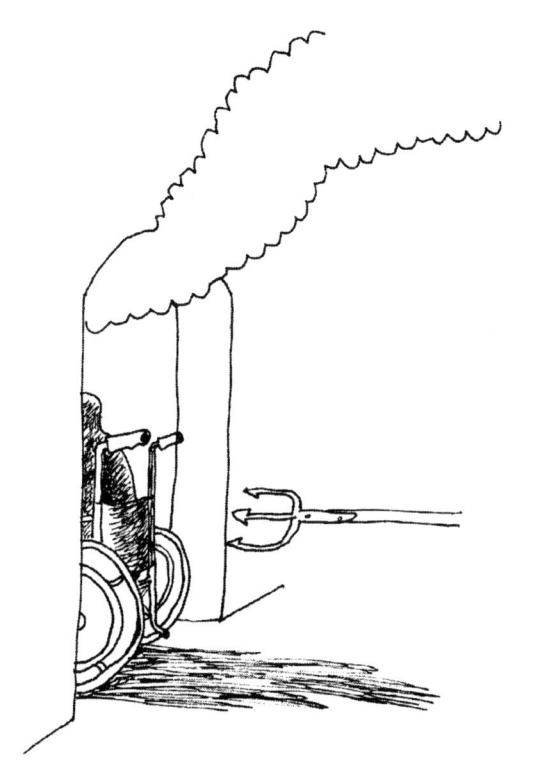

Cloud-access denied: all routes lead down.

Other books by Christopher Day:

Building with Heart (Green Books, Devon, 1990)

Places of the Soul (Thorsons / Harper Collins, London, 1990; 2nd. edition: Architectural Press Oxford, 2004)

A Haven for Childhood (Starborn Books, Rhydwilym, Clynderwen, Dyfed, 1998)

Spirit & Place (Architectural Press, Oxford, 2002)

Consensus Design (Architectural Press, Oxford, 2003)

Environment and Children (Architectural Press, Oxford, 2007)